Law for **Doctors**

Wai-Ching Leung

MRCP(UK) MRCPCH MRCGP MRCPsych LLB LLM
Senior Registrar in Public Health Medicine
Epidemiology and Public Health
Newcastle City Health Trust
Westgate Road
Newcastle-upon-Tyne
NE4 6BE

This book has been supplied by Eisai
Limited and Janssen-Cilag Limited. The
opinions expressed are those of the
authors and do not reflect those of
Eisai Limited or Janssen-Cilag Limited.

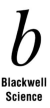

**Blackwell
Science**

©2000
Blackwell Science Ltd
Editorial Offices:
Osney Mead, Oxford OX2 0EL
25 John Street, London WC1N 2BS
23 Ainslie Place, Edinburgh EH3 6AJ
350 Main Street, Malden
  MA 02148-5018, USA
54 University Street, Carlton
  Victoria 3053, Australia
10, rue Casimir Delavigne
  75006 Paris, France

Other Editorial Offices:
Blackwell Wissenschafts-Verlag
  GmbH
Kurfürstendamm 57
10707 Berlin, Germany

Blackwell Science KK
MG Kodenmacho Building
7–10 Kodenmacho Nihombashi
Chuo-ku, Tokyo 104, Japan

First published 2000
Reprinted 2000

Set by Jayvee, Trivandrum, India
Printed and bound in Great Britain
at the Alden Press Ltd,
Oxford and Northampton

The Blackwell Science logo is a
trade mark of Blackwell Science Ltd,
registered at the United Kingdom
Trade Marks Registry

DISTRIBUTORS

Marston Book Services Ltd
PO Box 269
Abingdon, Oxon OX14 4YN
(*Orders*: Tel: 01235 465500
          Fax: 01235 465555)

USA
Blackwell Science, Inc.
Commerce Place
350 Main Street
Malden, MA 02148-5018
(*Orders*: Tel: 800 759 6102
          781 388 8250
          Fax: 781 388 8255)

Canada
Login Brothers Book Company
324 Saulteaux Crescent
Winnipeg, Manitoba R3J 3T2
(*Orders*: Tel: 204 837 2987)

Australia
Blackwell Science Pty Ltd
54 University Street
Carlton, Victoria 3053
(*Orders*: Tel: 3 9347 0300
          Fax: 3 9347 5001)

A catalogue record for this title
is available from the British Library

ISBN 0-632-05243-0

Library of Congress
Cataloging-in-publication Data
Leung, Wai-Ching.
  Law for doctors / Wai-Ching Leung.
    p. cm.
  ISBN 0-632-05243-0
  1. Medical laws and legislation—
  United Kingdom. I. Title.
  KF3821 .L47 2000
  344.73'041—dc21   00-020659

For further information on
Blackwell Science, visit our website:
www.blackwell-science.com

Contents

Preface

It is more important than ever for doctors and other health professionals to know about the basic theory and practical aspects of law which affect them. With increasing public expectations of the health service, medical litigation and complaints about the health service have been on the increase. The NHS structural reforms in recent years have produced important changes for health professionals as employees. There have been significant developments in the law concerning treatment of the mentally ill, patients' access to medical information and confidentiality. These issues affect all doctors and health professionals.

The General Medical Council recognized the importance of these aspects of law in the undergraduate curriculum in its document 'Tomorrow's doctor' (1993). Not only are students expected to be assessed on these areas in the new curriculum, but they need to know how to apply them to their work from their first day in their house jobs.

Currently, all books on these topics are large comprehensive textbooks of a theoretical nature. They are written in complex legal language, are highly referenced and are inaccessible to the average health professional and manager. They are also theoretical, and health professionals often find it difficult to apply the theory in practice. Moreover, many of them concentrate on one specialized topic (e.g. medical negligence) but exclude other important relevant topics (e.g. employment issues, the role of professional bodies, etc.).

There is therefore a need for a book on law that is relevant to doctors and other health professionals. This book covers the major areas of legal issues which doctors and other health professionals may encounter in their professional lives. Issues of theoretical interests only are avoided. It illustrates basic principles using examples familiar to them, focuses only on areas relevant to their practice, and highlights practical issues and good practice. Complex legal terms are avoided and legal references are kept to the minimum. Case histories which are familiar to health professionals are used to illustrate the issues.

The book is in three parts. The first part deals with the relationship between the health professionals and patients. The second part deals with various legal settings in which doctors' actions may be challenged. The third part deals with practical procedures which the health professional may encounter.

Wai-Ching Leung
November 1999

Part 1
Health Professionals and Patients

Chapter 1 – **Consent to medical treatment**

Read the following case histories and decide whether the medical treatment given by the doctors was legal.

Case 1

A woman presented with anaemia and her general practitioner (GP) decided that blood tests were required to determine the cause of her anaemia. The GP explained why blood tests were needed and had ready the necessary equipment for taking blood. He neither asked the patient to sign a consent form nor obtained explicit verbal agreement from her that she consented to have blood taken. However, the patient held out her arm and co-operated fully in the blood-taking procedure.

Case 2

A 42-year-old man was admitted to hospital for an inguinal hernia operation. The consultant surgeon saw the patient in a business ward round and explained the operation in detail; the patient verbally agreed to the operation. However, the house officer forgot to ask the patient to sign the consent form after the ward round. The consultant surgeon operated on the patient and only discovered the absence of a written consent form afterwards.

Had the consultant surgeon acted illegally? What should he do?

Case 3

A 37-year-old woman was placed on the waiting list for a hysterectomy for heavy periods by an inexperienced senior house officer in the out-patient department after discussion with his consultant. However, the senior house officer was not sufficiently knowledgeable to explain to the patient the nature of the operation. After she was admitted to the ward, he explained to her that his consultant would see her before the operation and asked her to sign a consent form. The patient readily complied. However, the consultant forgot to see the patient and only remembered his omission after her operation. The patient was surprised to hear that she would not be able to bear children again.

Case 4

A 38-year-old obese woman was admitted for laparoscopic sterilization. On admission, she appeared very nervous and asked the senior house officer whether she could still become pregnant after the operation and whether she would need a large abdominal incision. In order to allay the patient's anxiety, the senior house officer reassured the patient that she could not possibly become pregnant after the operation and that an abdominal incision would not be required. However, the laparoscopic procedure proved difficult and the patient required a mini-laparotomy procedure. Furthermore, although the operative techniques were excellent, the two ends of a severed Fallopian tube rejoined, and she became pregnant a year later. These are well known and accepted complications of a sterilization procedure.

Case 5

A 34-year-old woman presented with heavy periods and unexplained pelvic pain. She was admitted to hospital and consented to dilatation and curettage and diagnostic laparoscopy. During the procedure, numerous fibroids were found. The consultant gynaecologist felt that a total abdominal hysterectomy would be necessary in the near future and decided to proceed to hysterectomy immediately in order to save the patient from general anaesthesia for a second time.

General principles of consent

Patients who are treated by their doctors without legally valid consent may take two possible courses of action:
• action for battery; and
• action for negligence.
Negligence is discussed in detail in Chapter 9.

Practical differences between an action for battery and an action for negligence

Battery is intentional injuring (or even touching in a hostile manner) another person without his or her consent. Negligence is a breach of the professional's duty of care to the patient. To claim that a health professional was negligent, the patient must show that:
1 the professional breached a duty of care owed to the patient;
2 the patient suffered injury or damage; and
3 the injury was caused by the breach of duty.

From a practical point of view, there are two principal differences between suing for battery and suing for negligence. Firstly, in cases where patients claim that consent was invalid due to insufficient information given to them, a claim for negligence is possible, provided that the above three elements of negligence are present. However, the patient is unlikely to succeed in a claim for battery as long as the patient had been given the broad terms of the medical treatment (*Chatterton* v. *Gerson* 1981). Secondly, in an action for negligence, the patient is required to prove actual loss and damage and that the loss was foreseeably caused by the doctor's treatment. However, the patient is not required to prove actual loss and causation in an action for battery. Hence, a patient may succeed in an action for battery but fail in an action for negligence and vice versa.

The table on the opposite page compares and contrasts battery and negligence in relation to consent.

	Claim for battery	**Claim for negligence**
Nature	Either a criminal charge or a claim for compensation	A claim for compensation
Level of consent required to defend a claim	Broad terms of the treatment only	'Informed consent'
Need for patient to show actual loss or injury	No	Yes
Need for patient to show the loss was foreseeable	No	Yes

Battery

Legally, if a person injures or even touches another person deliberately and in a hostile manner without his or her consent, battery would have been committed. Battery may be both a criminal matter (leading to criminal prosecution) and a civil matter (allowing the victim to claim for compensation). As criminal battery requires ill intent, doctors are extremely rarely accused of criminal battery.

In the course of medical treatment, doctors often need to touch patients or even perform highly invasive procedures on them. Generally speaking, if legal consent has not been obtained from the patient, the patient may sue the doctor for battery in order to claim compensation. The patient need not prove that the doctor's treatment is below the normally accepted standard.

Consent required for defence against battery
Consent to medical treatment may be either expressed or implied. For minor medical procedures such as taking blood pressure or venepuncture, the mere co-operation with the procedure may be taken as legally valid implied consent. Hence, in case 1, neither verbal nor written consent is required. For more complicated or invasive medical procedures, expressed consent is required.

Legally, verbal and written consent are equally valid. The main difference is that evidence of patients' written consent can be produced much more easily than oral consent in court, which may be many years after the treatment has taken place. It is therefore important to obtain written consent from patients for invasive or major medical procedures, and the consent form should be carefully filed in the patient's records. In case 2, the oral consent obtained from the patient would be legally sufficient. However, producing satisfactory proof to the court on a later date that oral consent had been given may be practically difficult. After he had discovered the omission, the consultant should have asked the patient to sign a form stating that he had previously orally consented to the operation. Failing this, the consultant should document the oral consent in the medical records, together with the names of staff who had witnessed the oral consent.

Conversely, although a signed consent form usually constitutes a good defence against battery, this may not necessarily be the case if the doctor had not informed the patient of the broad nature of the medical procedure. Hence, in case 3, if the senior house officer had not even explained what hysterectomy was, the signed consent form alone would not constitute a good defence against battery.

On the other hand, if the broad nature of the procedure had been explained, the patient would not succeed in a claim for battery, even if the doctor had not fully explained the possible risks and complications resulting from the medical procedure (*Chatterton* v. *Gerson* 1981). However, the patient may still pursue a claim of negligence. Hence, in case 4, the patient would not succeed in a claim for battery as the nature of sterilization had been explained to her, even though the doctor had not explained the possibility of pregnancy and the possible need for a minilaparotomy. Even so, the patient might still succeed in a claim for negligence.

In case 5, the patient consented to dilatation and curettage and laparoscopy, but had not consented to hysterectomy. Although the doctor performed hysterectomy in order to save the patient from having to undergo general anaesthesia again, the procedure was not immediately necessary. Hence, the gynaecologist had not obtained legally valid consent from the patient and he could be sued for battery. He should have discussed the possibility of hysterectomy with the patient before the anaesthesia was administered. Failing this, he should have obtained consent from the patient following surgery and performed the hysterectomy at a later date.

Negligence

Informed consent is rooted in the concept of patients' self-determination—the patient's right to decide for him- or herself whether to accept treatment or not after taking into account all known facts. The general principles of negligence are discussed in Chapter 9. The principles of negligence applied to informed consent were hotly debated in the House of Lords in the well known case of *Sidaway* v. *Board of Governors of the Bethlem Royal Hospital* 1985 in which a neurosurgeon who proposed an operation on the patient's cervical vertebrae for recurrent pain did not inform her of the 1% risk of damage to the spinal cord. Generally speaking, to succeed in a claim for negligence due to lack of informed consent, the patient has to prove the following.

1 *Breach of a duty of disclosure owed to the patient.*
The Law Lords in the Sidaway case were divided as to how to determine whether the duty was breached. The four different approaches advocated by the four Law Lords were as follows.

(a) The Bolam test. The doctor has breached the duty of disclosure only if no responsible body of medical opinion would have withheld the information from the patient.

(b) The 'prudent patient' approach. The doctor must disclose all available information to the patient unless to do so would pose a serious threat to the patient's psychological health.

(c) The 'judge's decision' approach. The judge may decide that a doctor should have disclosed certain important information about potential serious side-effects, even if there is a responsible body of medical opinion who would not have disclosed the information to the patient. This was adopted in *Smith* v. *Tunbridge Wells Area Health Authority* 1984.

(d) The 'subjective patient test'. After explaining the general nature of the procedure, the doctor may wait for the patient to enquire about the general risks which should be obvious, unless the risks are very serious or very specific. If the patient does not ask any questions, it may be assumed that the patient trusts the doctor's judgement. Hence, the duty to disclose particular information is increased if the patient asks direct questions. Indeed, if the doctor fails to answer a specific question truthfully, the consent might be considered to have been fraudulently obtained.

2 *Loss and damage suffered by the patient.*

3 *Causation.*

The test usually adopted by the court is whether a reasonable person, sharing the characteristics of the particular patient, would have declined to undergo the procedure, or whether the patient could have taken special precautions to avoid losses.

In case 4, the risk of pregnancy and the possibility of the need for a mini-laparotomy are well known, and the senior house officer should have answered the patient's specific questions truthfully. Hence, the court is likely to hold the doctor in breach of his duty. The patient might also convince the court that she would not have undergone the procedure if she had been informed of the risks.

Who can legally give consent?

Read the following case histories and decide whether the consent given was valid.

Case 6

A 65-year-old woman was admitted to a surgical ward with a perforated duodenal ulcer. The surgeons arranged for an emergency repair operation. The patient's husband, seeing that his wife was in pain, offered to sign the consent form for his wife.

Case 7

A 34-year-old man was brought unconscious to the accident and emergency department by his wife on a Saturday night after a fight at a pub. A left-sided extradural haematoma was diagnosed.

How may valid consent be obtained for evacuation of the haematoma?

1 Any competent individual over 16 years can give consent to or refuse medical treatment.

2 Anyone with parental responsibility for a child under 18 years can give consent to medical treatment on behalf of the child.

3 No other persons (e.g. spouses, relatives or close friends) can legally give consent to the medical treatment on behalf of another person. Hence, in case 6, the husband cannot legally consent to the operation on behalf of his wife.

Capacity to consent

In general, all adults should be assumed to be competent to consent to or refuse medical treatment unless shown otherwise. Possible reasons why a person may lack capacity to consent to or refuse medical treatment include:
- minors (those under 16 years);
- physical illness (e.g. unconsciousness or drowsiness);
- mental disorder (including mental illness and mental handicap); and
- undue influence by others.

Emergency or life-saving treatment

English common law allows doctors to give emergency or life-saving treatments to their patients if it is in their best interests and the necessary consent cannot be obtained practically in the time available (e.g. if the patient is unconscious). However, this only applies to emergency treatments which are absolutely necessary.

   Hence, in case 7, the doctor could legally evacuate the extradural haematoma without oral or written consent from the patient.

Children and young people

Case 8
A 17-year-old boy with severe learning disabilities and a mental age of 3 years was admitted for an inguinal hernia repair. As the boy could not understand the nature of the operation, his mother signed the consent form on his behalf.

   Was the consent legally valid? Would the answer have been the same had the boy been 22 years old?

Case 9
A 17-year-old boy was admitted for an operation to correct bat ears. Although the patient was very keen to have the operation, both his parents objected to it.

   Is it legal for the doctor to operate with the boy's consent?

Case 10

A 16-year-old girl was admitted for tonsillectomy. Her parents were not available, and she signed the consent form for the operation.

Case 11

A 15-year-old girl asked her GP for a prescription for postcoital contraception. In spite of persuasion by the GP to discuss the matter with her parents, the girl refused to do so. The doctor prescribed the postcoital contraception without informing the girl's parents.

Case 12

An 8-year-old boy was admitted with a history suggesting acute appendicitis. The surgeons decided to perform an appendicectomy. Unfortunately, the child's parents were at work, and the surgeons asked him to sign the consent form himself.

Case 13

A 5-year-old boy was seen in the accident and emergency department with severe left-sided testicular pain. A surgeon saw the child and rapidly diagnosed torsion of the left testis; he recommended an emergency operation. However, the boy's parents were uneducated and superstitious and believed that the best course of action would be to take the child to a spiritual healer. In spite of the surgeon's careful explanation and warning that the child's life was in danger, the parents refused to give consent to the operation.
How may legally valid consent be obtained?

Case 14

A 4-year-old boy was seen with glue ears and conductive hearing loss. The ear, nose and throat (ENT) consultant considered tonsillectomy, adenoidectomy and insertion of grommets to be essential. Although the child's mother gave consent to the treatment, his father strongly objected.
Can the consultant proceed with the treatment?

Children under 18 years

The Children Act 1989 defines a child as a person under the age of 18 years. However, the Family Law Reform Act 1969, section 8 covers children over the age of 16 years. Hence, children under 16 years and those between the ages of 16 and 18 years should be considered separately.

Children between the ages of 16 and 18 years

Under the Children Act 1989, those with parental responsibility can give valid consent for children until the age of majority (18 years). However, under section 8 of the Family Law Reform Act 1969, competent children over the age of 16 years can give effective consent to any surgical or medical treatment, and it is not necessary to obtain any consent for it from the child's parents. Hence, a competent child's consent can generally override the wishes of those with parental responsibility.

Therefore, if the child is competent, either the child or one of those with parental responsibility can give legally valid consent. If they are in conflict, the child's wishes override those of the person with parental responsibility. However, if the child is incompetent, the parent can still give legally valid consent.

In case 8, since the child is under the age of 18 years, a person with parental responsibility can give legally valid consent to the inguinal hernia repair. As the child has a mental age of 3 years, he would be incompetent to consent to his own treatment. Had the patient been 22 years old, the Children Act 1989 would no longer apply, and his parents could not give legally valid consent for the operation. In fact, no one could give such consent.

In case 9, however, the boy was over the age of 16 years and was competent. Hence, he could legally consent to his own treatment. His decision would override that of his parents.

In case 10, the girl was over the age of 16 years and could give her own consent to treatment.

Children under the age of 16 years

Generally speaking, therapeutic medical treatment for children under the age of 16 years requires consent from one person with parental responsibility for the child. This consent is valid even if the child refuses treatment. An exception is non-therapeutic treatment such as sterilization, which requires consent from the High Court.

Before the Gillick case (*Gillick* v. *West Norfolk and Wisbech Area Health Authority*) in 1986, it was generally believed that consent from at least one parent was required for any treatment for a child under 16 years, and that treatment could not be given at the request of the child without the parent's consent. Mrs Gillick sought an assurance from the West Norfolk and Wisbech Area Health Authority that no contraceptive advice or treatment would be given to any of her daughters while they were under 16 years without her knowledge and consent, which the area health authority refused. The House of Lords held that a girl under 16 years had the legal capacity to consent to medical examination and treatment, including contraceptive treatment, if she had sufficient maturity and intelligence to understand the nature and implications of the proposed treatment. The parental right and responsibility to control a child derived from parental duty, which existed only when it was required for the child's benefit and protection. The extent and duration of this responsibility depended on the degree of intelligence and understanding of the child in question, and a judgement of what was best for the welfare of the child. The House of Lords held that doctors may be a better judge of the medical advice and treatment in exceptional cases, if necessary even without the knowledge of the parents. The determination of 'Gillick competence' is largely a matter for the doctor.

Thus, a child under 16 years who is able to understand the broad nature of a particular treatment has a right to consent to that treatment, and this cannot be overridden by parental responsibility.

In case 11, if the girl was able to understand the broad nature of postcoital contraception and the possible complications, she could legally consent to receiving the treatment, even if her parents objected. However, it would be good practice for the GP to involve the parents as far as possible.

On the other hand, those with parental responsibility can override the wishes of a child who is 'Gillick competent' by consenting to treatment which the child is refusing (*Re W (a minor)* (1992) and *Re K, W and H (minors)* (1993)).

In case 12, it is unlikely that an 8-year-old boy would have the capacity to understand the nature of appendicectomy and consent to it. Hence, the written consent from the boy is unlikely to be legally valid. The surgeons should have tried to contact his parents urgently. Failing this, they could have operated on the child on the grounds of necessity, as his case was an emergency and the operation was potentially life-saving.

In case 13, the child's parents refused to give consent to the treatment and the child was incompetent to give consent. However, as the treatment was urgent and life-saving, the surgeons should have acted in the best interests of the child and treated the child regardless. For less urgent treatment, a 'specific issue order' under the Children Act 1989, section 8 may be applied for to determine whether the child should have the medical treatment contemplated. In practice, it is advisable to ask an independent senior doctor to document the need for immediate treatment. If the parents insisted on removing the child, an emergency child protection order under the Children Act could be applied for.

In case 14, as the mother has parental responsibility for the child, her consent to treatment was legally valid and the ENT consultant could proceed with the treatment without fear of being sued for battery. It is clear from the Children Act 1989, section 2(7) and *Re R* (1991) that consent from one person with parental responsibility is sufficient, even if another person with parental responsibility objects. However, it would be good clinical practice to discuss the treatment with both parents in order to secure an agreement.

Mental handicap and mental illness

Case 15

A 50-year-old schizophrenic patient suffered from recurrent cholecystitis and required a cholecystectomy. He understood the nature of cholecystectomy which was explained to him by the surgeon, and believed that the operation would prevent the recurrent attacks of pain he had. However, he was grossly deluded in other respects, and believed that he was a messenger sent from God to rescue the world.

How may legally valid consent for cholecystectomy be obtained?

Case 16

A 36-year-old girl with severe learning disabilities and a mental age of 3 years became increasingly sexually active. Her parents felt that, without appropriate contraceptives, the girl would soon become pregnant and that this would be detrimental to the girl's mental health. After evaluating all contraceptive options, her parents and her doctor considered sterilization to be the most suitable method.

How may legally valid consent be obtained?

Case 17

A 23-year-old primigravid woman was admitted to the labour ward in the first stage of labour. Whilst being monitored, the fetus was suddenly found to be severely distressed. The obstetrician immediately recommended an emergency Caesarean section. In spite of careful explanation of the inevitability of fetal death if this were not carried out, the woman refused to give consent to the operation as she believed strongly in natural birth.

Can the obstetrician operate on the mother against her wishes?

Case 18

A 19-year-old girl with severe anorexia nervosa was admitted to a psychiatric ward with extremely low body weight, but refused to eat. The medical staff considered her condition to be critical, and that unless the girl was force-fed, she would soon die from starvation.

Can she be legally force-fed?

General principles

Whilst the psychiatric treatment for mentally disordered patients may be given under the Mental Health Act 1983, treatment for diseases which are not related to the mental disorder is governed by common law, and cannot be given under the Act. Psychiatric treatment for mentally disordered patients is discussed in Chapter 2. In this chapter, the treatment of physical conditions unrelated to the mental disorder is discussed.

The criteria for deciding whether a particular patient has the capacity to consent to a particular medical treatment are discussed in the case of *Re C* (1994). The three elements required are:

1 understanding and retaining treatment information;
2 believing it; and
3 weighing it in the balance to arrive at an informed choice.

It is important to note that capacity to consent must be assessed with a specific treatment proposal in mind, and that a patient may be competent to consent to a simple procedure but incompetent to consent to a more complicated procedure. In practical terms, the capacity to consent must be assessed when the treatment is proposed, and that assessment must be fully documented. Hence, the fact that a patient is grossly deluded does not necessarily imply that he or she cannot consent to any medical treatment.

In case 15, the patient appeared to understand the nature and purpose of cholecystectomy, as well as believing in its value. He appeared to be able to make a choice. Hence, he had the capacity to consent to cholecystectomy, irrespective of the delusions he had in other areas.

In case 16, the girl had a mental age of 3 years and clearly did not have the capacity to consent to sterilization. Furthermore, she was chronologically above the age of 18 years, and therefore her parents could not consent on her behalf. The facts in case 16 are somewhat similar to those in *Re F* (1990). In *Re F*, the House of Lords acknowledged that nobody could legally give consent on the patient's behalf. It solved the dilemma by making an advance declaration that the performance of sterilization by medical staff on the patient would not be unlawful. Hence, in case 16, the parents would have to apply to the High Court for such a declaration.

In case 17, the patient believed in natural birth and refused to undergo an emergency Caesarean section. It is clear that she did not suffer from any form of mental disorder, and was competent to refuse the proposed Caesarean section. Another issue is the balancing of the interests of the mother and the fetus. A few similar cases have been heard before the courts recently, and it is now clear that the mother has the capacity to refuse treatment and that it would be unlawful for the obstetrician to force a Caesarean section on her.

Case 18 is somewhat controversial. The first question is whether anorexia nervosa is a mental disorder which may come under the Mental Health Act 1983. It has been accepted that anorexia nervosa could be a mental disorder. The second question is whether force-feeding is a treatment for the psychiatric condition, or a physical treatment unrelated to the underlying mental disorder. It was held in *South-West Hertfordshire Health Authority* v. *KB* (1994) that force-feeding was an integral treatment of anorexia nervosa and therefore could be given under section 63 of the Mental Health Act 1983.

Incompetence due to undue influence

Case 19

A 54-year-old Jehovah's Witness was admitted to hospital with severe haematemesis due to bleeding from a duodenal ulcer. The patient became increasingly shocked in spite of saline infusion and drug treatment. Although the doctor considered a blood transfusion essential to save her life, she resolutely refused blood transfusion due to her religious beliefs. However, her 30-year-old daughter agreed that her mother should be given a blood transfusion, and asked the medical staff to administer it.

Case 20

A 23-year-old woman suffered from postpartum haemorrhage and urgently required a blood transfusion. The woman agreed initially. Later, her mother, who was a Jehovah's Witness, arrived. After a private discussion with her mother, the patient refused to have the blood transfusion, and signed a paper to this effect.

Can the doctors legally administer a blood transfusion?

In case 19, the patient refused a blood transfusion due to her religious beliefs. As she was competent to refuse the proposed treatment, it would be unlawful for the doctors to administer the blood transfusion against her will. The patient's daughter's consent would not be legally valid.

In case 20, the patient appeared to have been unduly influenced by her mother in deciding to refuse the proposed blood transfusion. The facts in case 20 are somewhat similar to those in *Re T* (1993). In *Re T*, it was acknowledged that, in deciding about capacity, doctors need to be aware of the possibility of undue influence. If undue influence is found, the capacity of the patient to consent may be reduced, and the patient's refusal to treatment may be vitiated. This is especially true for refusal to medical treatment which may involve a risk to life or of irreparable damage to health. Hence, in case 20, the doctors could argue that the capacity of the patient to refuse treatment was reduced because of undue influence by her mother, and may decide to administer the blood transfusion in the patient's own best interests. In practical terms, the opinion of an independent senior doctor should be sought and documented.

Key points

The form of consent

• Consent may be implied or expressed.
• Implied consent may be sufficient for minor procedures. Expressed consent is required for major or invasive procedures.
• Oral and written consent are equally valid in law. However, practically, it would be much easier to convince a court that consent had been given if it was written.
• It is important that doctors file and document all consent to treatment safely.

Battery and negligence

- Patients who are treated without legally valid consent may sue the doctor for (a) battery and (b) negligence.
- The practical differences between a claim of battery and negligence are:
  (a) a patient may succeed in a case of negligence, but is unlikely to succeed in a case of battery for alleged failure on the part of the doctor to disclose adequate information, as long as the broad nature of the treatment was explained; and
  (b) the patient needs to prove loss and causation for negligence, but not for battery.

How much information about the proposed treatment should be given to patients?

- The precise legal criteria are still unclear. However, patients should be given sufficient information to make an informed decision about whether or not to accept the treatment.
- If the patient asks specific questions about potential complications, he or she should be answered truthfully as far as possible.
- The information given to the patient should be documented in the medical records as far as possible.

Who can give legally valid consent?

- Any competent persons (i.e. persons with capacity to consent) over 16 years can give legally valid consent for their own treatment.
- Those with parental responsibility can give legally valid consent for children under 18 years.
- No other persons (e.g. relatives or close friends) can give legally valid consent to medical treatment.

Who has capacity to consent?

- All persons over 16 years of age are presumed to have the capacity to consent unless shown otherwise.
- Reasons for lack of capacity may include:
  (a) children under 16 years;
  (b) temporary or permanent physical disabilities (e.g. unconsciousness or drowsiness);
  (c) mental disorder (e.g. mental illness or mental handicap); and
  (d) undue influence from others.

Emergency or life-saving treatments

• Doctors may give essential emergency or life-saving treatments in the best interests of the patient without consent if such consent cannot be obtained practically.

Children under the age of 18 years

Children between the ages of 16 and 18 years

• Either the children, if they are competent, or those with parental responsibility can give consent to medical treatment.
• If the child is competent, his or her decisions override the decisions of those with parental responsibility.

Children under the age of 16 years

• All non-therapeutic treatments (e.g. sterilization) must be authorized by the High Court.
• Children under the age of 16 years may still give legally valid consent if they are 'Gillick competent', i.e. if they have sufficient maturity and intelligence to understand the nature and implications of the proposed treatment. (However, doctors should always try to persuade children to involve their parents in their treatment.)

Mental handicap and mental illness

• For mentally retarded adults over 18 years, it may be that nobody can give legally valid consent for their treatment. For non-urgent treatment, applications can be made to the courts for a declaration that such treatment without consent would not be unlawful.
• For patients detained under the Mental Health Act 1983, only treatments related to the mental disorder may be given under the Act. Other treatments must be given under common law.
• The capacity of mentally disordered patients to consent to medical treatment must be assessed with a particular treatment proposal in mind. A patient may have the capacity to consent to one treatment but at the same time lack the capacity to consent to another.
• The criteria for capacity to consent to medical treatment are:
  (a) understanding and retaining treatment information;
  (b) believing it; and
  (c) weighing it in the balance to arrive at a choice.
• The assessment of the capacity to consent to a particular treatment must be carefully documented.

Incompetence due to undue influence

• Occasionally, a patient may lack capacity to consent to or refuse a treatment because of undue influence by another person.
• This may be particularly important if refusal of treatment may involve a risk to life or irreparable damage to health.
• The medical staff should treat the patient in the patient's best interests should his or her capacity be reduced due to undue influence.

References

Chatterton v. *Gerson* [1981] QB 432.
Gillick v. *West Norfolk and Wisbech Area Health Authority* [1986] AC 112.
Sidaway v. *Board of Governors of the Bethlem Royal Hospital* [1985] AC 871.
Smith v. *Tunbridge Wells Area Health Authority* [1984] 5 Med LR 334.
South-West Hertfordshire Health Authority v. *KB* [1994] 2 FCR 1051.
Re C (adult: refusal of treatment) [1994] 1 WLR 290.
Re F (mental patient: sterilization) [1990] 2 AC 1.
Re K, W and H (minors) (medical treatment) [1993] 1 FLR 854.
Re R [1991] 4 All ER 177.
Re T (adult: refusal of treatment) [1993] Fam 95.
Re W (a minor) (medical treatment: court jurisdiction) [1992] 4 All ER 627.

Chapter 2 – **Treatment of mentally ill patients**

Introduction

People who are mentally ill may give rise to a number of legal problems: whether a third party may enforce a contract agreed by the mentally ill person, how society should deal with crimes committed by them and whether they should be allowed to administer their own properties or estates. The most important issue, however, is in which situations patients with mental health problems can be legally treated against their will. It is important to the patients themselves: inappropriate powers given to doctors may result in infringement of their autonomy and civil liberty, but inadequate powers may result in inadequate treatment of their illnesses. It is important to the health professionals, as they need to protect themselves legally as well as acting in the patients' best interests. It is important to the public, as a small proportion of untreated mentally ill patients may pose a danger to the public.

Since 1983, the Mental Health Act has dealt with the law relating to the assessment and treatment of mentally ill patients. The Mental Health Act 1983 starts on the basis that if a patient's condition is not serious enough to require hospital admission, it would not be justified to impose compulsory assessment and treatment. It has rapidly become out-dated, as both the health professionals and the Government consider that treatment of the mentally disordered should be mainly carried out in the community. Hence, the Mental Health Act 1983 no longer fits with the current patterns of service provision. In July 1998, the Government appointed a study team to undertake a root and branch review of the out-dated Mental Health Act 1983 to support the new national mental health strategy for England, and to develop a legislative framework for mental health care into the next millennium. The draft proposals of the review were published in April 1999 and have been presented to Ministers. The Green Paper 'Reform of the Mental Health Act 1983, Proposals for Consultation' was published in November 1999. Although it is likely that most of the proposals will be passed in Parliament in the near future, details may be subjected to change. The new proposals aim to ensure greater flexibility for compulsory care and treatment to be provided outside the hospital. The purpose of this chapter is to outline the main differences between the Mental Health Act 1983 and the new proposals, and some general principles which health professionals should adhere to in managing patients with mental health problems.

Key principles

Health professionals face a dilemma if patients with mental health problems and limited insight into their condition refuse treatment. On the one hand, the patient's autonomy and civil liberty need to be respected, and consent should be obtained before treatment is given. On the other hand, inaction may lead to further deterioration of the patient's condition, and may not be in the patient's best interests. Further, the health and safety of the patient and other people may be put at risk. Hence, a legal framework is needed to guide the health professionals and to protect patients.

The key principles of the Mental Health Act 1983 are mainly to balance autonomy of the patient and the health and safety of the patient and the public. Patients should be treated and cared for in such a way as to promote the greatest practical degree of self-determination and personal responsibility, consistent with their needs and wishes. Self-determination was given even greater emphasis in the proposals of the Steering Committee, but was toned down in the Green Paper. The guiding principles for the new Mental Health Act include the following.

• Informal care and treatment should always be considered before compulsory powers are introduced.

• Participation: service users should be involved as far as practical in their treatment.

• The safety of both the individual patient and the public is of key importance in deciding whether compulsory powers should be imposed.

• If patients are treated under compulsory powers, care and treatment should take place in the least restrictive setting consistent with the interests of the patient and the safety of the public.

Other principles endorsed by the Green Paper include the following.

• Non-discrimination: the principles which govern mental health care should be similar to those governing physical health.

• Least restrictive alternative: service users should be provided with treatment in the least invasive manner and least restrictive environment compatible with the delivery of safe and effective care.

• Reciprocity: society is obliged to provide high-quality services for those on whom it imposes compulsion.

Definition of mental disorder

The definition of mental disorder under the Mental Health Act 1983 is complicated, yet unclear. For admission for assessment under sections 2 or 4 or for removal to a place of safety under section 136, the patient should be suffering from some 'mental disorder'. However, for compulsory admission for treatment (section 3), the patient must have one of the four specific forms of mental disorder:

1 'mental illness';
2 'severe mental impairment';

3 'psychopathic disorder'; or

4 'mental impairment'.

Further, for compulsory admission for treatment, the disorder must be of the major type (i.e. not mental impairment or a psychopathic disorder) if the treatment is unlikely to improve the patient's condition. The exact definitions of terms such as 'mental illness' and 'severe mental impairment', etc. are not given. Several categories of mental disorder are explicitly excluded: sexual deviance, dependence on drugs or alcohol, promiscuity and other forms of immoral conduct.

This definition gives rise to the issue of the treatment of those with learning disability only. Patients with a learning disability do not have the capacity to consent to being admitted and treated, and yet they do not actively object. It is debatable whether they come under the definition of the Mental Health Act 1983. Traditionally, such patients are not 'sectioned'. Indeed, if formal Mental Health Act procedures had to be applied to all patients with a learning disability, many more resources would be required. The recent *Bournewood* case illustrated this legislative gap for those with a learning disability. In the *Bournewood* case, the Court of Appeal held that it was unlawful to admit an autistic adult to a psychiatric ward on an informal basis. Although the patient did not raise objections, he lacked capacity to consent to admission. If this ruling had stood, there would have been immense resource implications as there would have been insufficient mental health staff to place every patient who lacked capacity, including those with severe learning disability and dementia, under the Mental Health Act. The House of Lords overturned the decision in June 1998, so that it would not be unlawful to admit such patients informally.

Under the draft proposals, mental disorder is broadly defined as 'any disability or disorder of mind or brain whether permanent or temporary which results in an impairment or disturbance of mental functioning'. The term 'psychopathic disorder' is no longer used, although the term 'personality disorder' is retained. The express exclusion of alcohol and drug misuse is retained; sexual deviance is changed to 'disorders of sexual preference'; the express exclusion of promiscuity or other immoral conduct was felt unnecessary given the social changes since 1983. However, even patients with the diagnosis of one of these excluded categories would still be regarded as having a mental disorder under the new Act if they have a secondary diagnosis of another mental disorder.

Although the definition of 'mental disorder' is broadly defined under the new proposals, the criteria for compulsory assessment or treatment have become more stringent (Table 2.1). The clinical need for assessment and treatment after taking into account the risk, capacity and the best interests of the patient is given more emphasis than the formal psychiatric diagnosis of the patient.

Table 2.1

	Mental Health Act 1983	**Draft proposals of Mental Health Act review**
Definition of mental disorder	For sections 2 and 4, no specific definition For section 3, must be one of the four forms: mental illness, severe mental impairment, psychopathic disorder, mental impairment	Any disability or disorder of mind or brain whether permanent or temporary which results in an impairment or disturbance of mental functioning
	Explicitly excludes substance abuse, sexual deviance, drug or alcohol dependence, promiscuity or other immoral conduct	Explicitly excludes drug or alcohol misuse and disorders of sexual preference
Formal assessment (non-emergency)	Only in hospital	In hospital or community
	Application from two doctors (one specially approved), one approved social worker (or nearest relative)	Application from one approved doctor and other approved health professional
	Criteria: 1 Patient should be admitted in the interests of his or her own health or safety, or with a view to the protection of other persons 2 Patient suffers from a mental dis-order of a nature or degree that warrants detention in hospital for a period of assessment	Criteria: 1 Patient ought to be assessed in the interests of his or her own health and safety, or with a view to the protection of others 2 Adequate assessment cannot be conducted in the absence of compulsory power
	Assessment: observation as to whether compulsory treatment is needed	Assessment: assess capacity, risk, diagnosis, agreed care, treatment plan, community care need
	Valid for: 28 days	Valid for: 7 days
	Disposal: professionals may apply for compulsory treatment if necessary	Disposal: professionals need to apply to independent tribunal for provisional treatment order which lasts for 21 days
Emergency powers	*In hospitals (sections 5(2), 5(4))* One doctor—72 hours One registered nurse—6 hours *In community (section 4)* One doctor and one approved social worker (or nearest relative)—72 hours *In public place (section 136)* By police—72 hours	*In hospitals* Nurses with relevant specialist training—24 hours *In community* One mental health professional and one doctor—24 hours *In public place* By police—24 hours

Continued on p. 22

	Mental Health Act 1983	Draft proposals of Mental Health Act review
Compulsory treatment order	Application by one approved social worker (or nearest relative), one approved doctor, and one other doctor Criteria: 1 Presence of mental illness, severe mental impairment, psychopathic disorder or mental impairment of a nature or degree which makes it appropriate to receive treatment; 2 (if psychopathic disorder or mental impairment), treatment is likely to alleviate or prevent deterioration of the condition; and 3 treatment is necessary for the health and safety of the patient or others Place: in hospital Valid for: 6 months	Application by clinical supervisor to new specialist tribunal Criteria (according to model with test if capacity): 1 Presence of mental disorder, of a nature or degree that requires care and treatment under clinical supervision; 2 care and treatment plan proposed is the least restrictive alternative; consistent with safe and effective care; 3 care and treatment plan is in the patient's best interests; 4 (a) (if patient has no capacity) treatment is necessary for the health and safety of the patient or for the protection of others; (b) (if patient has capacity) there is substantial risk of serious harm to the health and safety of the patient, to the safety of other persons, and there is medical treatment available for the patient's mental disorder from which he or she is likely to benefit Place: in hospital or community Valid for: 6 months
Treatment with special safeguards	*Treatment requiring consent and second opinion (section 57)* • Neurosurgical procedures which destroy brain tissue • Hormone implantation to reduce male sexual drive *Treatment requiring consent or second opinion (section 58)* • Administration of drugs (if over 3 months) • ECT *Emergency* Consent or second opinion not required if immediately necessary to prevent serious deterioration of patient's condition	*Treatment requiring consent and tribunal approval* • Neurosurgical procedures • Hormone implantation to reduce male sexual drive *ECT, polypharmacy (3 or more drugs from same BNF class)* • (With capacity) cannot be given against patient's will • (Without capacity) express approval from tribunal must be obtained *All treatments* Initially approved by tribunal. Treatments after 2 months need to be reviewed by medical member of tribunal *Emergency* Medication can be given as before, but needs to be reported to the tribunal. ECT cannot be given without consent or tribunal's prior approval
The tribunal	*Mental Health Review Tribunal* Composition: medical, legal, and lay member	*New specialist tribunal* Composition: medical, legal, and someone with experience in mental health services; input from psychiatrists

Continued on p. 23

Mental Health Act 1983	**Draft proposals of Mental Health Act review**
Role: to decide whether the patient should be discharged	Role:
	1 Decide whether compulsion was appropriate in terms of the diagnosis, capacity and risk;
Frequency of involvement: section 2—patient may appeal within 14 days of section	2 if so, decide whether this should be in hospital or a community setting; and
section 3—patient may appeal once in the first 6 months, once in the second 6 months, and thereafter once every year	3 approve the care and treatment plan
	Frequency of involvement:
	Compulsory treatment:
	• to authorize the treatment initially
	• patient may appeal to the tribunal after 3 months

BNF, British National Formulary; ECT, electroconvulsive therapy.

General procedures for compulsory assessment and treatment

Under the Mental Health Act 1983, an approved social worker or the nearest relative of the patient may make the application for compulsory assessment and treatment. In practice, it is almost always the approved social worker who makes the application, as the nearest relative usually feels uneasy in making such applications. Compulsory assessment or treatment (sections 2 or 3) needs to be authorized by two doctors, one of whom must be specially approved.

The perceived problems of these procedures are that an approved social worker may not be familiar with the patient, and that a social worker may not be immediately available. It is often difficult to arrange for two doctors to assess the patient. Further, the hospital may not necessarily be an appropriate place to assess or treat the patient.

Under the new proposals, one admission route would replace the several distinct procedures in the 1983 Act. Under the draft proposals, it is recommended that an approved mental health professional may make the application. Such a health professional need not necessarily be a social worker. He or she may be a community psychiatric nurse who knows the patient better. However, this point is subject to consultation at the time of writing. The theoretical powers of the nearest relative to apply for admission are removed. As in the 1983 Act, compulsory assessment must be supported by two doctors, at least one of whom must have specialist training in psychiatry. However, the order will only last for up to 7 days initially. The main purpose of this period is to thoroughly assess the patient's condition, to prepare an outline care and treatment programme and to apply in writing to an independent reviewer for a 'provisional treatment order'. The independent reviewer may accept the application and grant a 21-day provisional order or call for a full tribunal hearing to be brought forward. Before the provisional treatment order is granted, only treatments which are emergency, life-saving or necessary to prevent deterioration or alleviate suffering may be given without consent. The provisional treatment order applies both in hospital and in the community. The maximum period of assessment and provisional treatment order combined is 28 days.

The criteria for compulsory assessment are slightly more stringent under the draft proposals. The proposals state that adequate assessment cannot be carried out in the absence of compulsory power. Once a compulsory assessment order is applied for, the draft proposals recommend that the following factors should be assessed by a multidisciplinary care team in order to apply for a provisional treatment order:
• the patient's capacity;
• the patient's mental (and physical?) condition;
• the risk in terms of both the seriousness of the feared harm and the likelihood of its occurrence or reoccurrence;
• a proposed care and treatment plan;
• the patient's community care needs; and
• the person's social and family circumstances.

Under the new proposals, if compulsory treatment is considered necessary, an application should be made to the new specialist tribunal (which replaces the old Mental Health Review Tribunal) to hold a full hearing. The care team needs to demonstrate that a further period of compulsory care is justified. If the tribunal decides that further compulsory care and treatment are justified, it can then decide whether such compulsory care and treatment should take place in hospital or in the community. The initial maximum period of such an order is 6 months. The composition of the new tribunal is still under consultation, but will include a legal Chair, a member with experience of the mental health service, and input from psychiatrists.

The criteria for a compulsory treatment order will be more stringent than those under the Mental Health Act 1983. The expert committee recommends that the capacity of the patient should be fully taken into account, in accordance with the common law. However, the Government believes that this may introduce differentiated risk thresholds for those with and without capacity, and may not fully protect the safety of individual patients and the public. The two models under consultation are detailed below.

1 *Model with a capacity test* (favoured by the initial Steering Committee):
  (a) the presence of mental disorder;
  (b) the mental disorder is of a nature or degree that requires care and treatment under supervision of specialist mental health services;
  (c) the proposed care and treatment plan is the least restrictive and invasive alternative available consistent with safe and effective care;
  (d) the care and treatment plan constitutes treatment in the patient's best interests;
  (e) (for patients who lack capacity), it is necessary for the health or safety of the patient or for the protection of others from serious harm that the patient be subject to such a care and treatment plan, and that such a plan cannot be implemented unless the patient is compelled under this section; and

(f) (for patients who have capacity), there is a substantial risk of serious harm to the health or safety of the patient or to the safety of other persons or of the patient being seriously exploited if he or she remains untreated, and there is medical treatment available for the mental disorder from which the patient is likely to benefit.

2 *Model without a capacity test* (put forward as an alternative in the Green Paper):

(a) the presence of mental disorder;

(b) the mental disorder is of a nature or degree that requires care and treatment under supervision of specialist mental health services;

(c) the proposed care and treatment cannot be implemented without the use of compulsory powers; and

(d) the treatment plan is necessary for (i) the health and safety of the patient (including issues relating to welfare and self-harm); (ii) the protection of others from serious harm; or (iii) the protection of the patient from serious exploitation.

The emphasis of the first model is on the 'autonomy' of the patient, whilst the emphasis of the second model is on the health and safety of the patient and the safety of the public.

If a compulsory treatment order is applied in the community, the order could:

• stipulate the place of residence;

• define the proposed care and treatment plan;

• confer an obligation on the patient to allow access and to be present for scheduled visits by identified caseworkers;

• impose a duty on health and social services to comply with arrangements set out in the care plans; and

• stipulate the consequences of non-compliance (e.g. power to enter premises or to convey the patient to hospital).

Capacity and the patient's 'best interests'

Capacity and the patient's 'best interests' are two important concepts in the Steering Committee's draft proposals, although they are much less significant in the alternative model put forward by the Government.

Capacity

The fundamental reason why treatment needs to be imposed on patients is that patients lack capacity to make the decision for themselves. Hence, the assessment of capacity is essential if the principles of non-discrimination and respecting the patients' autonomy are to be achieved. The assessment of capacity is not explicitly mentioned in the Mental Health Act 1983, but has been given much emphasis in the draft proposals.

Although the concept of capacity is important, it is not easy to assess in practice. Consent to different types of treatment requires different levels of capacity. The patient's condition may fluctuate from day to day, and there is inevitably a subjective element in the assessment of capacity.

The definition of capacity is still not finalized, and a test of capacity is under development. However, a provisional definition adopted from the Law Commission in the draft proposal is:

1 a person is deemed to have capacity until proven otherwise; and
2 a person may be deemed to lack capacity if:
   (a) he is unable to understand or retain the information relevant to taking the decision; or
   (b) although he can understand the relevant information, he is prevented by his mental disability from using that information to arrive at a choice.

Best interests

Ethically, if a treatment is to be imposed on a patient, it must be considered to be in the best interests of the patient. Although this criterion is not made explicit in the Mental Health Act 1983, it is given prominence in the recent mental health review draft proposals for compulsory treatment. What constitutes the best interests of the patient is debatable. It may mean either what the health professional would consider appropriate for the patient, or what the patient would be presumed to wish if he had capacity. It is also difficult to decide on which basis the presumed wishes of the patient should be determined. The recent draft proposals adopted by the Law Commission emphasize the need to take into account:

• the ascertainable past and present wishes of the person concerned and the factors that person would consider if able to do so;
• the need to permit the person to participate as far as possible or to improve his or her ability to participate;
• the views of other people whom it is appropriate and practicable to consult about the person's wishes and feelings and what would be in the person's best interests; and
• whether the proposed treatment is the least invasive and restrictive alternative.

Treatments subject to special safeguards

In general, the law of consent dictates whether certain medical treatments can be given legally. For patients under compulsory treatment, treatment for mental illnesses may be given against their will. However, special safeguards exist for some treatments which are particularly invasive or irreversible. Under the Mental Health Act 1983, there are two special categories. The first category includes neurosurgical procedures that destroy brain tissue and hormone implantation to reduce male sexual drive. These treatments require both the patient's consent and the approval of a second-opinion doctor (section 57). The second category includes administration of drugs for more than 3 months and electroconvulsive therapy (ECT). These treatments require either the patient's consent or the approval of a second-opinion doctor (section 58). In an emergency, however, ECT may be given against the patient's wishes before the approval of the second-opinion doctor is obtained.

In the recent mental health review, the draft proposals suggested that safeguards should include the following.

1 Treatments requiring both consent and tribunal's approval:

    (a) neurosurgical procedures for mental disorders; and

    (b) hormone implantation to reduce male sexual drive.

2 Treatments requiring the patient's consent (if capacity is present) or the special approval of the tribunal (if capacity is lacking):

    (a) ECT;

    (b) polypharmacy (three or more drugs within the same British National Formulary (BNF) group); and

    (c) feeding contrary to the will of the patient.

The Steering Committee recommended that it should not be possible to give the second category of treatments against the will of a patient with capacity. Treatment of an incapacitated person would require the special approval of the tribunal. These recommendations are under consultation.

Proposals for managing dangerous people with severe personality disorder

Currently, persons who are convicted of criminal offences but are found to suffer from psychiatric disorders can be detained in mental hospitals (usually, but not necessarily, in secure units) under different sections of the Mental Health Act 1983. Under the current law, there is a lack of flexibility in the transfer of patients between prison and the mental health services. Patients convicted of a criminal offence cannot usually be transferred back to the prison services once orders under the Mental Health Act 1983 have been given.

A few well publicized cases of patients with severe personality disorder posing risks to the public prompted the Government to make proposals for managing them. It is estimated that there are about 2000 people in England and Wales who fall into this category, most of whom have committed serious crimes and are either in prison or in secure hospitals. However, under the current law, they must be discharged to the community after they have served their sentences or if they no longer fulfil the criteria for detention in secure hospitals. However, they may remain dangerous. The interests of the patients as individuals and the public must be carefully balanced.

Two options are put forward in the Green Paper. Both rely on the development of new and more rigorous procedures for assessing risk associated with the presence of severe personality disorder. There are two objectives for these proposals: (i) to ensure that dangerous severely personality disordered people are kept in detention for as long as they pose a high risk; and (ii) to manage them in a way that provides better opportunities to deal with the consequences of their disorder.

The first option would be to improve arrangements in both prisons and the health service, and to introduce changes in the law based on the current framework of criminal and mental health law. Severely personality disordered people would not be released from prison or hospital whilst they continued to present a risk to the public. Any individual who had been convicted of a criminal offence and who was subject to a sentence of imprisonment would be held in prison. Anyone else would be held in a health service facility. The second option is to introduce an entirely new legal framework to provide powers for the indeterminate detention of dangerous, severely personality disordered people in both criminal and civil proceedings. Those detained under the new orders would be managed either in secure hospitals or in prisons. The location for detention would be based on the risk that the person represented and their therapeutic needs, rather than whether they had been convicted of an offence.

Case 1

The warden of a university hall of residence reported to a GP that a 20-year-old student had been behaving strangely for 2 days and was found to be carrying a knife. When the GP visited the student, he was extremely agitated and complained that all students in the university were spying on him using electronic means. He threatened to 'get them first' with the knife. The GP considered admission to hospital essential, but the patient refused.

What should the GP do?

Case 2

A 40-year-old woman had been diagnosed with schizophrenia 10 years previously and had been stabilized on depot medication. She lived in a warden-controlled hostel for mentally ill people. However, she had started to refuse medication 3 months earlier and had become withdrawn. She appeared to have auditory hallucinations and threatened to leave the hostel on several occasions. The GP visited but the patient refused to take medication or to remain in the hostel.

What should the GP do?

Case 3

A 25-year-old man was seen in the accident and emergency department after an overdose of aspirin. The psychiatrist assessed him and considered him to be suicidal, and the man agreed to be admitted to the psychiatric ward. However, 12h after admission, he refused to remain on the ward. The staff nurse in charge considered him to be at risk, but the psychiatrist was not immediately available.

What should the staff nurse do?

Case 4

A 23-year-old man had a long history of violent and antisocial behaviour and had been diagnosed with borderline personality disorder. He had previously been treated with major tranquillizers as well as with individual and group therapy, which had a limited effect on his behaviour. He lived with his 54-year-old mother in rented accommodation. He had been admitted to the psychiatric ward for assessment a few days earlier, as his mother noted that he had become more violent in the previous few days and found it difficult to cope with him. The psychiatrist found him unpredictable and irritable, and considered it unsuitable for him to live with his mother for the time being. After analysing the options available, the psychiatrist suggested that he remain in the ward for a combination of drug and psychotherapy treatment, although staff had reservations about the effectiveness of the proposed treatment. The patient understood and had good insight into his condition, but refused to remain in the hospital.

What should the psychiatrist do?

Case 5

A 35-year-old man with chronic paranoia and pathological jealousy was admitted to the psychiatric ward informally after threatening his wife with a knife. He had a chronic belief that his wife was unfaithful to him and that she was plotting against him. He had been treated with various antipsychotic drugs for many years, and the psychiatrists did not feel that any treatment would be effective. However, they considered that the safety of his wife would be at considerable risk if he was not admitted. Two days later, the patient insisted on leaving the ward so that he could 'sort his wife out'.

What should the psychiatrist do?

Case 6

A 30-year-old woman was admitted to the psychiatric ward under a compulsory assessment order after an overdose. She was found to be extremely depressed with very serious suicidal intent. The consultant psychiatrist considered that she should receive ECT immediately. The patient appeared to have insight into her illness. She agreed to take antidepressants but refused ECT treatment.

Should the psychiatrist administer ECT against her will?

Case 7

A 26-year-old man was admitted to the psychiatric ward with major psychotic symptoms under a compulsory treatment order. He developed severe right-sided abdominal pain whilst in the ward, and the surgeon on call diagnosed acute appen-dicitis. However, the patient refused to undergo appendicectomy despite careful explanation by the psychiatrist, the surgeon and his wife. The reason for his refusal was unclear, but was likely to be related to his delusions. The surgeon considered perfor-ation of his appendix imminent if appendicectomy was not performed immediately.

What should the surgeon and the psychiatrist do?

Analysis of the case histories

The case histories are analysed separately under the Mental Health Act 1983 and under the new mental health review proposals.

Case 1

Mental Health Act 1983

The patient clearly had an acute episode of psychosis and required admission to hospital immediately. If a second doctor (i.e. a section 12-approved psychiatrist) is available, an application can be made under section 2 for an assessment order. The approved duty social worker and the second doctor should be requested to assess the patient. An application could be made if it was agreed that the patient suffered from a form of mental disorder which warranted detention in hospital for assessment, and that he should be admitted for his own health and safety. This order would last for 28 days. If a second doctor is not available, the GP and the approved duty social worker can make an application for emergency admission under section 4. This order would last for 72 h. An application for compulsory assessment should be made under section 2 within this time. The application under section 2 would require the assessment by the approved social worker and two doctors (at least one of them section 12 approved).

Green Paper for Mental Health Act review

Under the draft proposals, the GP and an approved mental health professional (e.g. community psychiatric nurse or social worker) can make an application for emergency admission. This would last for 24 h, and an order for formal assess-ment should be made within this time. An approved doctor and an approved mental health professional (e.g. mental health nurse or social worker) should assess the patient and make the application for formal assessment. They need to be satisfied that the patient has a mental disorder and should be assessed in the interests of his own health and safety. They also need to be satisfied that adequate assessment cannot be made without compulsive power. This order would last for 7 days, during which the diagnosis, capacity and risks of the patient should be assessed and the treatment plan and community care needs should be agreed on by the mental health team. An independent reviewer would review the case, and a provisional treatment order lasting a maximum of 21 days may be granted. Care and treatment during this period may be given either in the hospital or in the community. If a compulsory treatment order is considered essential, an application should be made to the new specialist tribunal.

Case 2

Mental Health Act 1983

Under the Mental Health Act 1983, the patient could not be detained against her will in the community (e.g. in the hostel). If it was deemed necessary for the patient to be detained compulsorily for assessment or treatment, this should take place in hospital. In this case, she could be admitted to hospital compulsorily either for assessment (under section 2) or for treatment (under section 3). For either section, an approved social worker and two doctors should make the application. If the social worker and doctors thought they did not know the patient well enough, they should apply for compulsory assessment. However, they could apply for compulsory treatment if they considered that her illness was of a severity requiring treatment for her own health and safety.

Green Paper for Mental Health Act review

Under the draft proposals, an application could be made for compulsory assessment either in hospital or in the hostel. From the information given, it would appear that assessment in the hostel would be more appropriate. An approved psychiatrist and another approved mental health professional could make the application. This order would last for 7 days. Within 7 days, an independent reviewer may grant a provisional treatment order for 21 days. After this period of time, compulsory treatment may only be given after a full hearing by the new specialist tribunal.

Case 3

Mental Health Act 1983

If a patient admitted informally refused to remain on the ward, the mental health nurse could detain the patient for 6h under section 5(4) if the nurse believed that the patient should be detained for his or her own health and safety or for the safety of others. During this time, the duty doctor must assess the patient. If the doctor also agreed, an application under section 5(2) could be made which would last for 72h. An application for compulsory assessment (section 2) or compulsory treatment (section 3) must be made within the 72h if further detention of the patient is required.

Green Paper for Mental Health Act review

Under the draft proposals, any approved mental health professional (e.g. a registered mental health nurse) could make an application to detain patients who are already in hospital for 24h. An application for compulsory assessment or treatment must be made during this period if further detention of the patient is warranted.

Case 4

The issue is whether an application for compulsory treatment could be made. It will be seen that the final outcome is similar under the Mental Health Act 1983 and the Green Paper proposals.

Mental Health Act 1983

The patient suffered from a severe personality disorder. The issue is whether the patient could be admitted under section 3 for compulsory treatment. Psychopathic disorders are explicitly included as mental disorders under the Mental Health Act 1983. For mental illnesses and severe mental impairment, section 3 may be applied for if admission for treatment is in the best interests of the patient's health and safety or for the protection of others. However, there is an additional criterion for psychopathic disorder or mental impairment: treatment must be likely to alleviate or prevent deterioration of the condition. It appears that the treatment in this case would not alleviate the patient's condition, although the psychiatrist might argue that treatment may prevent deterioration of the condition. Hence, it is doubtful whether the patient could be treated under section 3.

Green Paper for Mental Health Act review

The outcome would depend on whether the criteria which enter the legislation in future are those with the capacity test or those without the capacity test. Assuming that the criteria with the capacity test are used, the first and second criteria do not pose difficulties. However, it would be difficult to argue that the proposed treatment (treatment in the ward, which is unlikely to be effective) would be in the patient's best interests. Further, it appears that the patient has capacity. Hence, in addition to the criterion that there is substantial risk of serious harm to the health and safety of the patient or to the safety of other persons, the psychiatrist must also be satisfied that there is medical treatment available for his mental disorder from which he is likely to benefit.

Hence, under both the Mental Health Act 1983 and the new draft proposals, it is doubtful whether application for compulsory treatment would be successful.

Case 5

Again, the issue is whether an application for compulsory treatment could be made. It will be seen that the final outcome is different under the Mental Health Act 1983 and the Green Paper proposals.

Mental Health Act 1983

The patient clearly has a serious mental illness, and it could be argued that compulsory detention for treatment is necessary for the safety of his wife. For mental illness, the criterion of 'treatability' does not apply. Hence, an application for compulsory treatment under section 3 is possible.

Green Paper for Mental Health Act review

The outcome would depend on whether the criteria which enter the legislation in future are those with the capacity test or those without the capacity test. If the model with the capacity test is used, it would be difficult to satisfy the third and fourth criteria for compulsory treatment. For the third criterion, it would be difficult to show that detention in hospital would be in the patient's best interests. For the fourth criterion, assuming that the patient has capacity, it is necessary to show that there is medical treatment available for his mental disorder from which he is likely to benefit. Hence, a successful application for compulsory treatment would be unlikely. If the model without the capacity test is used, then all the criteria are satisfied. The last criterion is satisfied as compulsory treatment is needed for the protection of others from serious harm. An application for a treatment order would be successful.

Case 6

It will be seen that the final outcome may be different under the Mental Health Act 1983 and the proposals in the Green Paper.

Mental Health Act 1983

It is clear that a successful application for compulsory treatment under section 3 could be made. Under section 58 of the Act, the patient may be given ECT against her will if a second independent doctor approved this treatment. Furthermore, under section 62, the patient may be given emergency ECT before this approval was obtained.

Green Paper for Mental Health Act review

Under the proposals of the Steering Committee, it would not be possible to administer ECT as an emergency before approval from the tribunal is obtained. Furthermore, if the patient was judged to have capacity, ECT could not be given against her will, irrespective of the tribunal's opinion. However, the Steering Committee's recommendations are still under consultation.

Case 7

Mental Health Act 1983

The power of the Mental Health Act 1983 to administer treatment against the patient's will is only restricted to treatment for the underlying mental disorder. It does not apply to treatment of physical illnesses unrelated to the mental disorder. Hence, it would not be possible to perform the appendicectomy under the Mental Health Act 1983. However, appendicectomy is clearly immediately necessary to save the patient's life, and is in the patient's best interests. The patient was not mentally competent to make a decision about the treatment.

Under these circumstances, it would be possible under common law to proceed to appendicectomy without consent. It would be good clinical practice, however, to obtain and document the opinion of another consultant surgeon. It is also essential to make full notes of the reasons for the decision.

Green Paper for Mental Health Act review

There are no new powers in the new draft proposals for health professionals to give treatment for physical illnesses which are not in the agreed treatment plan approved by the tribunal. Hence, as under the Mental Health Act 1983, the surgeon should perform appendicectomy under common law.

Key points

• Mental health law governs the treatment of mental health patients against their will.
• It is important for patients, the health professionals and the public. For the patients, it balances their best interests and their self-determination. For the health professionals, it provides clear guidance of what they should do. For the public, it serves to protect them from the minority of mental health patients who may represent a danger.
• The Mental Health Act 1983 will be replaced by new proposals, probably from 2001.
• The guiding principles in the new proposals include the consideration of informal care and treatment before using compulsory power, patients'

involvement, consideration for the safety of both the individual patient and the public, and caring for the patient in the least restrictive setting.

• Under the new proposals, a patient may be compulsorily treated in hospital or in the community.

• Whilst a patient is being compulsorily assessed, his or her capacity, mental condition, risk, family and social circumstances, and community care needs must be assessed within the period, and a care and treatment plan proposed.

• Capacity and the patient's best interests become important concepts. Under the Steering Committee's recommendations, the patient's capacity and best interests must be assessed and taken into account in the application for a compulsory treatment order.

References

Department of Health. Draft outline proposals by Scoping Study Committee.

Department of Health Review of Mental Health Act 1983. London: Department of Health, April 1999.

Department of Health (Green Paper) Reform of Mental Health Act 1983—Proposals for Consultation. London: Department of Health, November 1999.

R v. *Bournewood Community and Mental Health NHS Trust ex parte L.* House of Lords judgement, 25 June 1998.

Chapter 3 – **Confidentiality**

Ethical basis

Keeping confidences of patients' information gained in the course of medical consultation has been an important part of health professionals' ethics for a long time. There are many ethical arguments in favour of confidentiality.

• If patients are not certain that the information divulged in a consultation will be kept confidential, they may be less willing to divulge sensitive information which may be important for the diagnosis and management.

• There is always an implied agreement between the doctor and the patient that information divulged in a medical consultation will be kept confidential.

• Not keeping confidences would be damaging to the patient's self-determination and privacy.

The largely ethics-based nature of confidentiality is nowadays reflected by the fact that professional bodies (e.g. General Medical Council (GMC) and United Kingdom Central Council for Nursing, Midwifery and Health Visiting (UKCC)) are heavily involved in issues relating to confidentiality.

Legal basis

The law on confidentiality has developed in a haphazard fashion, so that there is no unified legal source on confidentiality. Instead, the courts have interpreted various areas of law in such a way as to give some legal support to the ethical basis of confidentiality highlighted above.

What is breach of confidentiality?

Read the following case histories and decide whether there has been a breach of confidentiality by the health professional involved.

Case 1

After conducting a busy ward round, the gynaecology registrar discussed the patients' management plans with the nurse in charge. In the process, it was necessary to mention some sensitive information about the patients. This discussion took place within the earshot of several patients and visitors.

Case 2

On receipt of a positive pregnancy test of a patient, the GP attempted to telephone the patient. Unfortunately, the patient was out and the telephone was answered by the patient's friend. The GP informed the friend of the result, and asked the friend to pass on the message to the patient.

Case 3

A woman had just died of carcinoma of the cervix. Two years previously, the woman's GP gave her psychotherapy for recurrent depression. After several psychotherapy sessions, the GP came to believe that the depression was related to a termination of pregnancy which the woman had undergone many years earlier. The patient made it clear at the time that she did not wish anyone to know about the termination. After her funeral, the GP discussed the psychotherapy sessions with the patient's husband and children.

Case 4

A 60-year-old woman was recovering from a heart attack in a medical ward. She was found to be obese and the doctor referred her to a dietician for advice. Without previously seeking explicit consent from the patient, the physician invited the dietician to browse through the patient's medical records.

Case 5

In a hospital clinical meeting, a patient's medical history was presented and discussed. A handout with the patient's name, date of birth and clinical summary was also distributed, which participants could take away from the meeting. The audit meeting could have been attended by any health professionals in the hospital.

Case 6

A child was admitted to a paediatric ward with symptoms of unknown cause. A local newspaper heard about and became interested in the child's mysterious illness. A reporter approached the doctor involved, who proceeded to discuss the clinical details with the reporter without mentioning the child's name. Although the name of the child was not reported, many residents in the local village knew the identity of the child from other details such as age, race, school and other characteristics.

In general, all personal information divulged by a patient to a health professional should be treated confidentially and not passed to a third party. Most breaches of confidentiality by health professionals are committed inadvertently, and they may not even be aware of the breaches. Everyday examples include doctors and nurses discussing patients within the earshot of other patients and visitors. Hence, case 1 is an example of breach of confidentiality. Although few patients would take any legal action under these circumstances, all health professionals should take care to avoid such incidents.

Health professionals must not assume that the patient would consent to confidential information being passed to them via their friends and relatives. In case 2, the GP should have left a message for the patient to call the doctor back.

The health professional's duty of confidentiality continues after the patient's death. This principle has been endorsed both in the Declaration of Geneva and by the World Health Organization. In case 3, the GP's duty of confidentiality continues even after the patient's death, and he should not have discussed the termination of her pregnancy with her family. However, the health professional may assume that patients consent to disclosure of information to other health professionals involved in their care. No explicit consent is required to share information amongst the members of the health-care team involved in the patient's care. In case 4, the physician need not obtain explicit consent from the patient for disclosure of information to the dietician, unless the patient explicitly refuses consent.

On the other hand, the health professional must not assume that patients would consent to disclosure of information to other health professionals not involved in their care. In case 5, circulation of handouts with identifiable patient information amongst all health professionals in the hospital would be a frank breach of confidentiality. Similarly, it must not be assumed that patients would consent to disclosure of information to researchers or to publication of their clinical details in a medical journal. Hence, before any clinical data are passed on to a medical researcher, all data which might identify the patient must be removed. Nowadays, most major medical journals require explicit written consent from patients before publishing clinical case reports.

Breaches of confidentiality may occur if it can be reasonably expected that the patient may be identified from information divulged by the health professionals. This may occur even if the name of the patient is not disclosed. Hence, there appears to be a breach of confidentiality in case 6.

Exceptions to the general rule of confidentiality

Read the following case histories and decide whether disclosure of information by the health professional involved would be justified.

Case 7

A GP, Dr X, treated a 45-year-old man with recurrent back pain in his surgery, who needed to be off work for a significant period of time. Recently, Dr X had also started work as a part-time occupational health physician in a large company, where the patient also worked as a porter. The personnel manager of the company learnt that Dr X was the patient's usual GP, and asked him to submit a medical report. The personnel manager suggested that Dr X should compel the patient to sign a consent form under the threat that he would otherwise perform another examination in his new role as an occupational health physician, and the same report would be submitted to the personnel department anyway.
Should Dr X comply?

Case 8

A 76-year-old woman in a medical ward had just undergone bronchoscopy and was diagnosed as suffering from carcinoma of the bronchus with liver metastasis. Her only surviving relative was her husband. Before the house physician had a chance to talk to the patient, he was summoned to the ward by the ward nursing staff to see the patient's husband alone. The husband pressed the doctor to inform him of the diagnosis, and to promise not to inform the patient if she proved to have a terminal illness.

Should the house physician inform the patient's husband of the diagnosis and comply with his wishes?

Case 9

A 25-year-old woman was admitted to the gynaecology ward for a termination of pregnancy in England. After she was discharged, the following individuals learnt about her admission without her explicit consent:
- the secretary who typed up the discharge summary;
- the clerk who filed her notes;
- a clinical researcher who was carrying out research into the treatment of abortion;
- a social worker in the district; and
- the Chief Medical Officer of England and Wales.

Has there been a breach of confidentiality?

Case 10

A clinician informed the Consultant in Communicable Disease Control of two patients without their explicit consent:
- a case of newly diagnosed tuberculosis; and
- a case of newly diagnosed acquired immune deficiency syndrome (AIDS).

Has there been a breach of confidentiality?

Case 11

A GP was questioned by a policeman who was investigating a case of shoplifting the previous day. A young man was spotted shoplifting by a shopkeeper who attempted to detain him. A struggle followed, during which the young man's left arm was injured. However, he managed to escape before the police arrived. A passer-by witnessed the young man entering the GP's surgery, possibly to seek treatment for the injured arm. The policeman asked the GP to confirm that such a patient had visited him the day before, and to divulge the name, address and telephone number of the patient involved.

Should the GP give the relevant information to the police?

Case 12

A GP was asked by a policeman to supply details of one of his patients who was suspected to be a dangerous multiple murderer. The police had been investigating a series of murders thought to have been committed by a single person living locally. According to the evidence available, the police believed that the suspect had visited the GP the previous day. The GP remembered the patient distinctly, as he was a well known drug abuser and had been asking for benzodiazepines frequently. The patient was extremely agitated during his last visit. From the description given by the police, the GP was convinced that there was a grave risk that he might commit a serious crime again.

Should the GP give the relevant information to the police?

Case 13

A 29-year-old man was treated by a GP for minor facial injuries after he was assaulted by his acquaintance. Six months later, the acquaintance was prosecuted and the GP was asked to give evidence in court about his patient's injuries. In the course of giving evidence, the barrister for the defendant (the patient's acquaintance) asked the GP about the patient's sexual orientation. The doctor knew about the patient's homosexuality as he had advised him on several occasions about sexually transmitted diseases.

Should he answer the barrister's questions truthfully?

Case 14

A 39-year-old heavy goods vehicle driver had three epileptic attacks and a neurologist had started treatment with anticonvulsants. The patient was counselled by his GP, who advised him to inform the Driver and Vehicle Licensing Agency (DVLA). However, the patient refused to do so as his livelihood depended on his driving licence. Two weeks later, the epileptic attacks became more frequent and occurred in the daytime, often without prior warning. The patient was adamant that he would not inform the DVLA, and insisted that the GP should not do so either.

What should the GP do?

Case 15

A 24-year-old man diagnosed with borderline personality disorder was seen by a psychiatrist. In the course of the consultation, the patient informed the psychiatrist about a conspiracy to blow up a government building. The psychiatrist enquired in detail, and the patient appeared to be serious about the plan.

What should the psychiatrist do?

Case 16

A GP counselled a 15-year-old girl with emotional problems. In the course of the consultation, the patient informed the doctor about repeated sexual abuse by her stepfather, whom the patient was still living with. There were no other children living with him. However, the girl was adamant that the GP should not inform anyone else about this.

What should the GP do?

Case 17

A 34-year-old man had recently been diagnosed as HIV positive. His GP informed him about the risks to his wife, encouraged him to discuss the diagnosis frankly with her, and offered to see the couple together. However, the patient refused to discuss the matter with his wife and asked the doctor not to tell her. Furthermore, the patient did not appear keen to use condoms. His wife was also a patient of the doctor. The man said that he had no sexual relationships with anyone other than his wife.

What should the GP do?

Case 18

A 50-year-old locum gynaecology registrar had recently been diagnosed to be HIV positive, and it was thought that he might have had the disease for 3 years. As there was a chance, albeit minimal, that the patients on whom he had operated could be infected, lookback exercises were planned to screen all patients operated on by the gynaecologist within the last 3 years. However, this proved difficult as he had worked in over 25 different hospitals in the past 3 years. The media came to know about this issue and demanded that hospital managers release information about the doctor. They argued that this was necessary to preserve press freedom and to allow a public debate on the matter. The medical directors and hospital managers felt that releasing limited information about the doctor to the public might allow more patients to come forward to be screened. It was clear that the gynaecologist was reluctant for this information to be released, although he did agree to sign a consent form for disclosure under emotional blackmail.

What should the medical directors and hospital managers do?

Although health professionals are under both a legal and a moral duty of confidentiality, exceptions to this obligation include:
1 when the patient gives consent;
2 when others need to know for the patient's care;
3 when there is a statutory duty (i.e. a duty required by Parliament);
4 when a warrant is issued by a circuit judge under the Police and Criminal Evidence Act 1984;
5 when explicit instructions are given by a judge in court; and
6 when the wider public's interest outweighs the interests of confidentiality.

Patient's consent

The most common justification for a health professional to divulge a patient's information to a third party is when it is done with the patient's explicit consent. It is important to document the patient's consent in a written consent form. If this is not practical, the patient's consent should be documented in his or her medical records. The patient's consent must be given voluntarily.

In case 7, the patient divulged the information to the doctor as a GP and did not anticipate that the doctor would become the occupational health physician of the company he worked for. Hence, there could not have been either implicit or explicit consent from the patient to divulge information to the personnel manager. If the doctor had submitted a report, it would have been a breach of confidentiality. Even if the doctor had been both a GP and an occupational health physician when the patient consulted him, he still could not divulge the information to the personnel manager unless he had clearly explained to the patient before the consultation of his duty to the company and of the possibility that he might have to submit a report. The personnel manager's suggestion to compel the patient to consent under the threat that a similar report would be submitted in any event after a second examination is highly inappropriate. Such consent would be given under duress and would not be legally valid.

Giving information to relatives

Relatives have no legal right to information without the patient's consent. Hence, it would be a breach of confidentiality to inform relatives about patients without their consent. It would be good clinical practice to see the relatives with the patient, and to seek the patient's prior permission to see his or her relatives, if possible.

In case 8, strictly speaking, it would be a breach of confidentiality for the house physician to see the patient's husband alone and inform him of the diagnosis without the patient's consent. It would be even more inappropriate to yield to the husband's demand to withhold the diagnosis from the patient. The correct approach would be to see the patient first, and then offer to see the couple jointly.

Those with a 'need to know' for patients' care

As stated previously, patients are implied to consent to the sharing of information amongst health professionals directly involved in their care, such as physiotherapists, dieticians, etc., unless they explicitly state otherwise.

However, there may be other staff who may need to have access to named-patient information. Examples include secretaries who type the discharge summaries, data clerks who enter information on a computer, and laboratory and radiology staff who participate in the investigation of the patient's illness. A social worker working in a child abuse case or with mental health patients may also need to have access to a patient's medical information. A doctor may wish to report a patient's unexpected reactions to drugs in order to improve drug safety.

Other staff may need to know about patients' confidential information, although the data may be made anonymous. Examples include public health doctors and health services managers who wish to analyse the health demands of the population and to carry out health service planning, clinical audit officers and medical researchers. Data could be given to this class of staff, but the data should be made available in a form such that the individual patients cannot be identified.

A 1996 Department of Health guidance has accepted that the 'need to know' exception to confidentiality exists. However, a European directive has made it clear that the information should be given in a form so that the patients cannot be identified.

In case 9, it is clear that the secretary who typed up the discharge summary and the clerk who filed the patient's notes need access to her records. Although the researcher would need to have some data, they may be given in a form such that the patient's identity is not revealed. The social worker in the district should be allowed access to information only if this is essential to the carrying out of his or her duties for this patient.

Statutory duties

There are areas of health care in which Parliament requires the health professionals to disclose information to the appropriate authorities. Under these circumstances, health professionals are obliged to disclose the information even if the patients object.

Examples of statutory duties to disclose confidential information include:
• notification of births and deaths under the Birth and Death Registration Acts;
• children born as a result of infertility treatment under the Human Fertilization and Embryology Act 1990;
• notice of terminations of pregnancies to be given to the relevant Chief Medical Officer under the Abortion Act 1967;
• treatment of drug addicts to be notified to the Home Office under the Misuse of Drugs Act (Notification of Supply to Addict) Regulation 1973;
• notifiable infectious diseases (e.g. tuberculosis, food poisoning and meningococcal diseases) to be notified to the district Consultant in Communicable Disease Control. HIV is not currently a notifiable disease.

Hence, in case 9, the Chief Medical Officer should be notified of the termination of pregnancy. In case 10, a case of tuberculosis should be notified to the Consultant in Communicable Disease Control, as it is a notifiable disease. However, HIV is currently not a notifiable disease, and consent should legally be sought from the patient. Alternatively, anonymous data may be provided to the Consultant in Communicable Disease Control for statistical analysis.

Enquiries from the police in their investigation of crime

Health professionals do not have a general legal duty to disclose confidential information to the police to help them in the investigation of crimes. Although the police may be able to obtain most evidence of crime by obtaining a warrant from a magistrate, they cannot obtain confidential health records using such a warrant. In exceptional circumstances, they may apply for a warrant from a circuit judge under the Police and Criminal Evidence Act 1984, section 9 and schedule 1 to obtain access to such confidential records.

However, there are exceptions. For example, the Road Traffic Act 1988 compels all citizens to provide the police with information at their request on the identity of drivers suspected of having committed a traffic offence.

Although health professionals may not be obliged by law to disclose confidential information which may help the police in their investigation of crime, they may choose to do so if they consider the public interest outweighs the importance of keeping confidences. Such circumstances may occur if the crime was very serious and if prevention or detection of the crime would be made much more difficult if the confidential information was not divulged to the police.

In case 11, there is no legal duty for the doctor to give the information to the police. The doctor might consider shoplifting not to be a serious enough offence to justify a breach of his patient's confidentiality.

Case 12 is in many ways similar to case 11, except that the crime involved was much more serious. Furthermore, the risk of the crime being committed again is much higher. Although there is no legal duty on the part of the doctor to inform the police, the doctor might consider it justified to breach the patient's confidentiality in order to prevent further serious crimes.

Explicit instructions from a judge in court

Health professionals are asked to give evidence for a variety of reasons. If they are called by a patient or a patient's lawyers, the patient would have given implied consent. However, if health professionals are not called by the patient, difficulties would arise if they were asked to divulge confidential information by the lawyers. Furthermore, the information sought may not be absolutely essential to the decision of the case. Whilst the communication between a lawyer and a client is 'privileged' and a lawyer is under no obligation to disclose it in court, communication between a doctor and a patient is not privileged.

The usual advice is that the doctor should inform the judge explicitly that answering the questions would involve a breach of medical confidentiality. Most judges would not require health professionals to answer the questions unless the information is critical to the decision of the case. However, if the judge explicitly instructs a health professional to give the information, this instruction must be obeyed or the health professional may face being held in contempt of court.

In case 13, the doctor was expecting to give evidence on the facial injuries of his patient, but not on his sexual orientation. The defence lawyer may have raised this question in order to use provocation as a defence. The doctor should explicitly inform the judge that answering the question would breach medical confidentiality, and wait for further instructions from the judge.

Wider public interests in disclosure outweigh the interests of confidentiality

As stated previously, it is in the public's interest for health professionals to keep confidences, as patients would otherwise be less willing to divulge sensitive information which may be important for diagnosis and management. However, on rare occasions, there may be competing public interest in disclosure which outweighs the interests of confidentiality. The balance between these two public interests can sometimes be difficult to judge.

Prevention of death or injury to others

One such competing public interest which may outweigh the interests of confidentiality is the prevention of death or injury to others. In balancing these two factors, health professionals have to judge the degree of risk of injury to others and the severity of the injuries should they occur. This is in accordance with the guidelines of the professional bodies. However, the final decision on individual cases rests with the health professionals themselves, and they must be able to justify their decisions if they are called to account for their actions.

In case 14, the doctor had to balance the public interest of confidentiality against the public interest of preventing road traffic accidents. The doctor might consider that the risk of accidents was significant as the frequency of the patient's epileptic attacks was increasing. The injuries to others could be fatal. Hence, the doctor should encourage the patient to report the illness to the DVLA himself. If the patient still refused, the doctor may choose to report the patient's illness himself.

In case 15, the doctor had to balance against the public interest of confidentiality the public interest of preventing a serious crime which may potentially severely injure a large number of people. Hence, the doctor may decide to give relevant information to the police. In a legal case, *R* v. *Egdell* 1990, the lawyers for a patient who was detained under the Mental Health Act 1983 instructed a psychiatrist to prepare a psychiatric report to be used in the Mental Health Review Tribunal. The psychiatrist found the patient to be extremely dangerous with a persistent interest in explosives. It was held that the psychiatrist was entitled to disclose his report to the Home Office against the patient's wishes.

Case 16 poses a difficult dilemma for the doctor. When the child first consulted the doctor, the doctor might not have expected the issue of child sexual abuse to be raised. Otherwise, the doctor should have warned the child that other agencies may need to be informed and involved. With the child's disclosure of sexual abuse, the doctor has to consider two issues: (i) the risks of further abuse to the child; and (ii) the risks of abuse to other children. The doctor may consider risks of abuse to other children unlikely, as no other children were living with the stepfather. However, the risks of further abuse to the child concerned remained. Under the Children Act 1989, the doctor had a duty to protect the child from abuse. Hence, the doctor may choose to inform Social Services in order to invoke the usual child protection procedures. It has been held in several legal cases recently that prevention of child abuse clearly justifies a breach of confidentiality.

Case 17 may prove to be even more difficult. The GP had to consider the risks to others if the patient did not inform his sexual partners of his disease and take appropriate precautions. It appears that the patient had no sexual partners other than his wife. Hence, the only issue to consider is the risk to his wife. The consequences of contracting the disease are very serious. Furthermore, as the GP also looked after the patient's wife, it would appear that he had a duty to give appropriate health advice to her. This would be difficult without disclosing confidential information about her husband.

The need for public debate, press freedom and patients' safety

It has sometimes been argued that the need for public debate and press freedom might justify a breach of confidentiality. In X v. Y 1988, a newspaper discovered that two doctors had been treated for AIDS through a hospital employee where the doctors were treated. The hospital attempted to obtain an injunction preventing the newspaper from disclosing the confidential information. The newspaper argued that disclosure was necessary to stimulate a public debate. Whilst recognizing the need for public debate, the court held that this need was outweighed by the guarantee of confidentiality which was necessary to ensure that AIDS sufferers were not discouraged from using the services.

As publicity concerning children who are made wards of court requires the court's permission, the courts have considered a number of cases in which the privacy of children had to be balanced against the public's need for debate. The factors which should be taken into account include what minimum information needs to be disclosed to stimulate a debate, and the harm to the children if the information is disclosed.

In case 18, the need to stimulate public debate and press freedom would not be adequate justification for disclosure of the doctor's confidential information, following X v. Y 1988. However, the argument that publicity might encourage more potentially infected patients to come forward to be screened may justify such disclosure. A similar incident had occurred in the past, and the doctor concerned had given permission for his name and condition to be disclosed. However, if the doctor had refused, the balancing of the need for confidentiality and patients' safety may have proven to be difficult.

Patients' redress for breach of confidentiality

The most frequent actions patients take if their confidentiality is breached are complaints:
• to the employers of health professionals;
• using the NHS complaints procedures; and
• to the professional bodies (e.g. GMC, UKCC).
Through these procedures, guilty health professionals may be appropriately punished and the chance of future similar incidents may be minimized. However, patients cannot obtain compensation through these procedures.

Very few patients actually take legal actions for breach of confidentiality. If they do, they may attempt to claim compensation for one or more of the following:
• breach of contract;
• medical negligence; or
• breach of a specific equitable obligation to keep a patient's information secret.

Key points

• All personal information divulged by a patient to a health professional should be treated confidentially and not passed to a third party.
• Unless authorized explicitly by the patient, this includes the patient's friends and relatives.
• The duty of confidentiality continues after the patient's death.
• Most breaches of confidentiality are inadvertent.
• Exceptions to the duty of confidentiality include:
  (a) patient's consent;
  (b) those with a need to know for the patient's care;
  (c) statutory duty (i.e. duty required by Parliament);
  (d) a warrant issued by a circuit judge under the Police and Criminal Evidence Act 1984;
  (e) explicit instructions from a judge in court; and
  (f) wider public's interest outweighs the interests of confidentiality.

References

R v. *Egdell* [1990] 1 All ER 835.
X v. *Y* [1988] 2 All ER 649.

Chapter 4 – **Access to personal medical information**

Up until the 1980s, patients had no common law general rights to see their own health records. The general arguments against patients seeing their health records are that they may not understand the technical language and that misunderstandings may occur in spite of careful explanation by the health professionals. It has been argued that these misunderstandings may sometimes be harmful to patients' physical or mental health. In recent years, it has been increasingly recognized that patients have the right to access their own medical records and that this might even improve communication between patients and health professionals. Patients' rights of access to their records have been recognized by several statutes which have been passed by Parliament. The Acts of Parliament which are directly relevant to health professionals are briefly summarized in the following table.

Act of Parliament	Types of health records applicable	Circumstances when patients may apply for access
Supreme Court Act 1981	Any health records	If the patient needs the information to take legal action for negligence
Data Protection Act 1984	Computerized records	At the request of the data subjects
Access to Medical Reports Act 1988	Reports supplied by a doctor for employment or insurance purposes	The subject of the report has a right to see the report before or up to 6 months after the report is sent
Access to Health Records Act 1990	Manual health records made since 1 November 1991	At the request of a patient, an authorized person, a parent or the personal representative of the deceased person

Safeguards are built into most of these statutes so that the data-holder may refuse access if the health professionals consider that access to records may be harmful to the physical or mental health of the patient.

Access to computerized and manual health records: the Data Protection Act 1984 and the Access to Health Records Act 1990

Read the following case histories.

Case 1

The medical records in a general practice have been partially computerized since 1986. Anna is a 35-year-old patient of the practice. Anna's father was suspected to have died of Huntington's chorea 20 years ago, but this was never positively confirmed. Anna's sister, Mary, is also a patient in the practice, and received genetic testing for the disease. However, as Mary does not get on well with Anna, she did not inform Anna of the results. Anna discovered that Mary's genetic test results would have been entered in Anna's own computerized records. As Anna's doctor refused to tell her of Mary's genetic test results for reasons of medical confidentiality, she decided to request access to her own medical records according to one of the statutes.

Does she have a right of access to her computerized medical records?

Case 2

Peter is 30 years old and has been diagnosed with a personality disorder. In the practice, doctors' notes are recorded manually, whilst general personal and health information, prescriptions and the notes made by nurses and dieticians are computerized. After an argument with the nurse, Peter requested that the practice manager allow him to see his computerized records. The nurse, who had made personal remarks about the patient in the computerized records, insisted that the patient should not be allowed access, using 'potential mental harm to the patient' as a reason. Both the doctor and the practice manager felt that the patient should be allowed access.

Who should decide whether to let Peter have access to his computerized medical records? In the event, Peter was refused access. What could he do?

Case 3

John is 45 years old and has presented with psychosomatic symptoms to various specialists in a hospital since 1984. He becomes increasingly dissatisfied with the treatments given by the specialists and decides to request access to his entire manual hospital medical records.

To whom should he make this request? Who should decide whether he should be given access? Does John have the right to access to the entire manual records?

When John was given a copy of the manual records, there were many technical terms he did not understand. Does he have a right to have the unintelligible terms explained to him? John also disagreed with several pieces of factual information in the notes. What could he do?

Case 4

An 8-year-old boy was referred to hospital by a GP for suspected appendicitis. After several days' observation, the boy was diagnosed with an appendix mass and an operation was performed several days later. The boy's parents were generally dissatisfied with the management and the explanations given by the surgeons and wished to request access to the child's medical notes.

Do they have a right of access to the notes? If so, to whom should they apply?

Case 5

A 15-year-old girl requested contraceptives from her GP, and insisted that her parents should not know about it. The doctor, having decided that the girl was Gillick competent, prescribed contraceptives as requested. The girl's mother suspected this and requested access to the manual records made by the GP under the Access to Health Records Act 1990.

Should the GP grant her access to her daughter's records?

Case 6

A 6-year-old girl presented with multiple bruises in the accident and emergency department. She was seen by a paediatrician who suspected child physical and sexual abuse. The child was admitted to the ward and was interviewed. The child then disclosed her father as the perpetrator of the abuse. A case conference was arranged. The girl's parents were informed of the suspected abuse, but the source of the information was withheld. In the meantime, the child's father applied to the NHS Trust for access to his daughter's manual medical records under the Access to Health Records Act 1990 to find out why he was suspected to be the perpetrator of the abuse.

Should the father be given access to the child's medical records?

Case 7

A 43-year-old woman had a termination of pregnancy in 1992 and made it clear to her GP that she did not wish anyone to know about it. The patient has recently died of carcinoma of the breast and her husband has requested access to her manual medical records under the Access to Health Records Act 1990.

Can he be refused access to the records?

Case 8

A 60-year-old woman was diagnosed with carcinoma of the breast, and the prognosis was considered to be poor. This was fully documented in a letter from a consultant surgeon to her GP. The GP did not inform the patient of the diagnosis, as he thought she was in a phase of denial and was not prepared to receive the news. The patient made an application under the Access to Health Records Act 1990 to see her manual medical records.

What should the doctor do?

Case 9

Mrs Smith is an 86-year-old physically frail lady who has been on a long-stay geriatric ward for over a year. Her only relative is her 56-year-old daughter, who visits Mrs Smith regularly. Her daughter has been increasingly dissatisfied with the inadequate explanations of her mother's condition, and suggested to her mother that she should apply for access to her notes. As Mrs Smith is illiterate, she signed an authorization letter for her daughter to have access to her medical records. Her daughter then made an application under the Access to Health Records Act 1990 to see her mother's notes.

Should her application be allowed?

The Data Protection Act 1984

The Data Protection Act 1984 is concerned with personal information held on computer. It provides general rules as well as rules on confidentiality and the rights of access by people on whom data are held.

The Act provides general rules about personal information held on computer: the persons holding the data must register under the Act; the information must be accurate; the information must be no more or no less detailed than required for the purpose for which it is held; and the information must not be stored for purposes other than those specified on the register.

The Act allows people on whom data are held to demand from the data-holder a copy of any data held on them within 40 days on payment of a fee. In general, the primary purpose is for them to check the accuracy of the information. When applied to health records, this allows patients to access their own health records. If the data-holder does not comply, the patient may apply to the courts to force the data-holder to release the data.

In practice, the computer data-holders in secondary care are mostly NHS Trusts, although the health authorities hold the contract minimum data set. In primary care, the computer data-holders are GPs, although the health authorities may hold some records such as those for cervical cytology call–recall.

Data Protection (Subject Access Modifications) (Health) Order 1987 applies to information about a person's physical or mental health held by, or originally held by, a health professional (including doctors, dentists, nurses, midwives, chemists, dieticians, osteopaths, etc.). It requires the data-holders (if they are not themselves health professionals) to consult a health professional who will decide whether to allow or refuse access to the information sought. The health professional need not be the person who originally recorded the information. The Order gives discretion to health professionals to refuse patients access to the information if:

1 this is likely to cause serious harm to the physical or mental health of the patient; or

2 access would breach the confidences of third parties. However, this only exempts the data-holder to disclose this part of the record. It also does not apply if the third person consents.

In case 1, Anna's application for access to her computerized records can be made to her GP, who is the data-holder. The doctor's dilemma is that disclosure would involve release of Mary's personal information, and Mary has not given consent for its disclosure to Anna. However, the doctor may (and should) refuse access to Mary's genetic test results on the grounds that access would breach the confidences of a third party. The doctor should give Anna access to data other than those related to Mary.

In case 2, access to computerized records should be made under the Data

Protection Act 1984. It is good clinical practice to consult the health professional who originally recorded the information about whether to allow access to the data and to come to a satisfactory agreement. However, although the practice nurse originally recorded the data requested, the data-holder was most likely to be the GP. The crucial test was who was registered as the data-holder under the Data Protection Act 1984. As the GP was both a data-holder and a relevant health professional, he could decide to allow the patient access to the data. Even if the practice manager were the data-holder, he or she would still need to consult a health professional (i.e. the doctor or the nurse). Hence, the practice manager could not make the final decision to allow or refuse access.

In any event, it would be inappropriate to use 'likely to cause serious harm to the physical or mental health of the patient' as a ground of refusal if the real issue was the personal remarks made by the nurse. This case demonstrates that it is most unwise to make personal remarks on a patient's records. If the doctor refused access to the information, the patient may apply to the courts for an order to force the doctor to comply with the request for access.

The Access to Health Records Act 1990

This Act covers manual health records made since 1 November 1991. Health records include information on the physical or mental health of a person recorded by or on behalf of a health professional in relation to the person's care. It includes records made by a wide variety of health professionals. However, it excludes records already covered by the Data Protection Act 1984.

Applications for access should be made to the record-holder. In practice, this would be the health authority or NHS Trust in secondary or tertiary care, and the GP in primary care. If the patient has not registered with a GP, application can be made to the relevant health authority.

Unless there is a specific ground for refusing access to information, the record-holder must allow access to the information within 21 days (for records made within 40 days of the application), or within 40 days (for records made more than 40 days before the application). To allow access to the information, the record-holder must allow the applicant to inspect the records, and to have a copy on payment of a fee. Terms unintelligible to the applicant must be explained. If the record-holder refuses to allow access within the specified time, the applicant may apply to the courts to force the record-holder to comply.

Whereas only people on whom data are held can apply under the Data Protection Act 1984, the following classes of people can apply under the Access to Health Records Act 1990:
• patients over the age of 16 years;
• patients under the age of 16 years who understand the nature of the application;

- those with parental responsibility for a child patient (only if the child consents, and it is in the best interests of the child);
- a person with written authorization from the patient;
- a person appointed by the courts to manage the affairs of an incompetent patient;
- the personal representative of a deceased patient (unless the patient has previously explicitly or implicitly refused consent); and
- anyone who may have a claim arising out of a patient's death (but only information relevant to the claim can be disclosed).

The record-holders, if they are not themselves appropriate health professionals, must consult the appropriate health professionals in order to find out whether applications for access should be allowed. The grounds for withholding information are:

- that the information would be likely to cause serious harm to the physical or mental health of the patient;
- that the information would be likely to cause serious harm to the physical or mental health of another person other than the patient;
- that the information would identify an informant (unless the informant consents to the application for access, or the informant is a health professional involved with the patient care);
- that the record was made before 1 November 1991; and
- that the record would show that an individual might have been born as a result of infertility treatment.

In case 3, John should apply in writing to the managers of the relevant NHS Trust for access to his notes. The managers should then contact the relevant clinicians to decide whether he should be given access. Under the Access to Health Records Act 1990, John is only entitled to have access to records made since 1 November 1991. However, in practice, most NHS Trusts usually allow access to the entire manual records. Ideally, the clinicians should arrange a time with John so that they can go through the notes with him, and explain any terms which he may not understand. If John disagreed with any factual information, he has a right under the Act to ask the NHS Trust as record-holders to correct the mistakes. After consulting with the clinicians, the NHS Trust should either correct the mistakes or make a note in the records of the patient's view of the mistakes.

In case 4, the parents have a right to access to the child's manual records, if the child consents and it is in the interests of the child. In this case, there was no evidence that the child would object, or that it was not in the child's interest to allow access. Hence, the parents should be given access. In fact, the parents' request probably reflected communication problems between the child and his parents and the health professionals, and the surgeons should have spent more time explaining the child's condition to the parents.

In case 5, the mother's application for access to her child's manual records should be refused, as the child had refused consent to her parents' access. Access under the Access to Health Records Act 1990 provides that those with parental responsibility should not be given access unless the child consents or is incapable of understanding the nature of the application.

In case 6, the father's application for access to the child's manual records should also be refused. Although it could be said that the child may not understand what is going on regarding access to the records, the Act provides that access may be refused if it is not in the best interests of the child. In this case, the health professionals may regard disclosing the child as the informant of the father's abuse may not be in the child's best interests.

In case 7, the Act allows the personal representative of the deceased to apply for access to the manual health records. However, if the patient had previously vetoed access to the applicant, this would be a reason to bar disclosure. In this case, the patient clearly did not wish her husband to know about her termination of pregnancy. Hence, her husband should be refused access to parts of the records which may reveal her previous termination of pregnancy. However, other parts of the records may be disclosed. The 1990 Act does not require the data-holder to inform the applicant that some information has been withheld.

In case 8, the doctor did not inform the patient of the diagnosis because he believed that the patient was in a phase of denial and was not prepared to hear the bad news. However, the fact that the patient applied for access to her notes probably meant that the doctor was wrong in his judgement, and that she had been eager to know about the diagnosis. The patient clearly had a right to apply for access to her manual records under the Access to Health Records Act 1990. In this case, it would be inappropriate for the doctor to bar access using 'the information would be likely to cause serious harm to the mental health of the patient' as the reason. The doctor should use this opportunity to spend more time with the patient and to discuss the diagnosis fully with her.

In case 9, the daughter of the patient had a right to apply for access to the manual medical records under the Access to Health Records Act 1990, as she had written authorization from the patient. There was no apparent reason why the daughter should be barred access. The doctors should use this opportunity to explain the patient's condition more fully to both the patient and her daughter.

Reports supplied by a doctor for employment or insurance purposes

Case 10

A teacher was provisionally offered a post at a school pending satisfactory clearance from the occupational health department. The teacher then disclosed in a staff health questionnaire that she had been treated for recurrent back pain. The occupational health department wished to ask for a report from the GP who had previously treated her back pain. The teacher wanted to see the report before it was sent to her employer.

What steps should the occupational health department take? What rights did the patient have to see the report? If she disagreed with some of the statements in the report what could she do?

Case 11

A 35-year-old man applied to be accepted for life insurance. After reading the initial questionnaire, the company decided to invite the man to be seen by a doctor who was specially commissioned by the company to provide a report for insurance purposes.

Did the man have a right to see the report before it was sent to the insurance company?

Case 12

A 45-year-old engineer for British Rail had been on sick leave for prolonged periods of time with back pain certified by his GP. The managers at British Rail heard informally from other workers that his sickness might not be genuine, and hence asked the occupational health physician to provide a report. The managers also asked the occupational health physician to interview some other employees who allegedly saw the engineer playing football whilst off sick with 'back pain'. After interviewing the employees and examining the patient, the occupational health physician wrote a report which strongly suggested that the patient's illness was not genuine. The patient insisted on seeing a copy of the report under the Access to Medical Reports Act 1988.

What should the occupational health physician do?

The Access to Medical Reports Act 1988

This Act applies to reports supplied for employment or insurance purposes by 'a medical practitioner who is or has been responsible for the clinical care of the individual'. This certainly includes reports by GPs and hospital doctors. It would appear that doctors who are commissioned purely to provide a report for employment or insurance purposes only are not covered. Whether reports written by occupational health physicians are covered is debatable, as occupational health physicians have a duty to protect the health of employees in the workplace.

Under the Act, those commissioning reports for employment or insurance purposes (i.e. employers and insurance companies) must first write to notify the subject about the report commissioned, inform the subject about his or her rights under the Act and obtain written consent from the subject. The subject may either choose to see the report before it is sent to the employers or insurers or choose not to see it.

If the patient chooses to see the report, the employer or insurance company must inform the doctor about this. If the patient does not arrange access, the doctor must wait for at least 21 days before sending off the report. If the patient sees the report, he or she may ask the doctor to amend parts of the report which he or she considers to be inaccurate. The doctor must either comply with the patient's wishes or append to the report a statement of the patient's view. The doctor must obtain written permission from the patient before sending off the report.

Patients who choose not to see the report should sign a statement to this effect. However, they may change their mind by writing to the doctor concerned. Even after the report has been sent, they may see the report for up to 6 months afterwards.

Doctors may refuse access to the report if:
• this is likely to cause serious harm to the physical or mental health of the individual seeking it, or to others;
• it would breach confidentiality of the doctor's informants; or
• it would disclose information about a third party.
Doctors refusing access to information must inform the subject that this is so.

In case 10, the GP's report to the teacher's employer is clearly covered by the Access to Medical Reports Act 1988. The employer should first seek written consent from the teacher and inform her of her right to access to the report before it is sent to the employer. If she disagreed with any statements in the report, she could ask her GP to amend it. The doctor would then need to either amend it as requested, or to append to the report a statement of the patient's view.

In case 11, the doctor was commissioned purely to provide a report for insurance purposes. As the Access to Medical Reports Act 1988 only covers reports supplied by a medical practitioner who is or has been responsible for the clinical care of the individual, the report is unlikely to be covered by the Act. Hence, the patient may not have a right to access to the report.

In case 12, the doctor is an occupational health physician, and it can be argued that he is or has been responsible for the clinical care of the patient. However, the doctor may still refuse the patient access to the part of the report related to the interviews of other employees, as access may breach the confidences of the doctor's informants.

Information needed to assess the strength of a legal claim: the Supreme Court Act 1981

For those who suspect that they have a legal claim but need further information to assess the strength of their case, this Act allows them to discover evidence they need to make their claim, and this may involve inspecting their medical records. This Act was particularly important before 1991 as it may have been the only way of discovering information. Arguably, it became less important when the Access to Health Records Act 1990 came into force.

The courts should be satisfied that some legal action is likely to follow if discovery is allowed, and that there is some chance of success. If patients do not know what they are looking for and are merely looking at their records in the hope that something will turn up, the courts would not allow patients to use this Act as a 'fishing expedition'.

If the courts are convinced by the health professionals that the patient's health may suffer if the records are disclosed, they may order the medical records to be disclosed to the patient's doctors or lawyers.

Key points

• There are no common law rights to access one's own medical records. The rights of access are given in different statutes passed since the 1980s.

• Access to computerized records by data subjects is governed by the Data Protection Act 1984, whilst access by the patient or other interested parties to manual medical records made since 1 November 1991 is governed by the Access to Health Records Act 1990.

• Access to medical reports made for employment or insurance purposes is governed by the Access to Medical Reports Act 1988.

• The discovery of medical reports in order to assess the strength of a legal claim under the Supreme Court Act 1981 has become less important.

• Safeguards are built into all these statutes to exempt health professionals from disclosing information if they consider that this would be harmful to the physical or mental health of the patient, or if the confidences of a third party would be breached.

Chapter 5 – **Abortion**

Abortion is an emotional and controversial issue. One argument in favour of abortion is that women have a right to control their bodies and hence they have a right to have abortions. An argument in favour of abortion put forward by many doctors is that, if abortions are illegal, many women will undergo illegal abortions carried out by unqualified people in a dangerous manner ('back-street abortion'). On the other hand, the argument against abortion is that life begins from conception or implantation, and that abortion would therefore constitute murder.

In England and Wales, the laws against abortion can be found in the Offences Against the Person Act 1861 and the Infant Life (Preservation) Act 1929. In brief, the Offences Against the Person Act 1861 prohibits causing a miscarriage (i.e. before 24 weeks of gestation), whereas the Infant Life (Preservation) Act 1929 prohibits the killing of a baby capable of being born alive (i.e. after 24 weeks of gestation). However, the Abortion Act 1967 provides defence against abortion as long as certain conditions are fulfilled, and the prescribed procedures are completed. The Human Fertilization and Embryology Act 1990 amended some of these conditions to be fulfilled.

In deciding whether a termination of pregnancy would be legal, the following questions must be asked.

1 Is it an 'abortion' legally?
2 Have the procedures prescribed in the Abortion Act 1967 been completed?
3 Is one of the conditions in the amended Abortion Act 1967 fulfilled?

Is it an 'abortion' legally?

Read the following case histories and decide whether there has been an 'abortion' legally.

Case 1

Thirty-six hours after an episode of unprotected sex, a 17-year-old girl requested post-coital contraception from her GP. He prescribed Schering PC4.

Was it necessary to follow the procedures in the Abortion Act 1967?

Case 2

A 24-year-old woman asked a gynaecologist to terminate her pregnancy as her last menstrual period was 7 weeks ago and her pregnancy test was positive. After detailed discussion with the patient, the doctor decided not to perform a surgical termination, but to prescribe the drug mifepristone (RU 486).

Was it necessary to follow the procedures in the Abortion Act 1967?

Case 3

A 32-year-old woman presented to a gynaecologist for infertility treatment. After treatment for 9 months, the woman became pregnant with quadruplets. The gynaecologist considered it unlikely that there would be any viable pregnancy unless three embryos were selectively killed in order to allow one embryo to develop. After this 'selective reduction' procedure, the dead embryos would simply be absorbed into the mother's body, and they would not be expelled from the uterus.

Was it necessary to follow the procedures in the Abortion Act 1967?

The crucial question is whether either the Offences Against the Person Act 1861 or the Infant Life (Preservation) Act 1929 has been contravened.

The Offences Against the Person Act 1861 makes it illegal for anyone to assist a woman with the intention of causing a miscarriage, whether or not the woman is in fact pregnant. It has been hotly debated whether the term 'miscarriage' should apply after fertilization or after implantation of the embryo in the uterus, and most agree that the term should apply after implantation. This is confirmed by the Human Fertilization and Embryology Act 1990, which confirms that a woman is not to be treated as carrying a child until the embryo has become implanted.

In case 1, prescription of the 'morning-after pill' causes failure of implantation after conception. Hence, this would not constitute a miscarriage and the procedures in the Abortion Act 1967 need not be followed. Similarly, the insertion of an intrauterine contraceptive device prevents implantation.

In case 2, prescription of mifepristone (RU 486) may dislodge an embryo implanted in the uterus. Hence, it would constitute a miscarriage and the procedures in the Abortion Act 1967 must be followed.

In selective reduction of multiple pregnancy, some of the embryos are killed to allow the other embryos to survive and develop. This is often performed for multiple pregnancy after infertility treatment. In selective reduction, the dead embryos are not expelled from the uterus, but are reabsorbed into the mother's body. Hence, whether case 3 constitutes a miscarriage depends on whether miscarriage is defined as expulsion of the embryo or the cessation of survival of the embryo. Most lawyers favour the latter definition. In any event, it is now made clear in the Human Fertilization and Embryology Act 1990 that selective reduction constitutes miscarriage and the procedures in the Abortion Act 1967 must be followed.

Have the procedures prescribed in the Abortion Act 1967 been completed?

The amended Abortion Act 1967 requires the following procedures to be completed.

1 *Medical opinion.*

   (a) Two qualified medical practitioners have formed an opinion in good faith that one of the conditions in the amended Abortion Act 1967 below is satisfied, and signed the prescribed certificate; or

(b) if one qualified medical practitioner has formed an opinion in good faith that an abortion is immediately necessary to save the mother's life or to prevent grave permanent injury to her physical and mental health, a second opinion is not necessary.

Although not required by law, it is good clinical practice for the prescribed certificate to be signed by the patient's GP and a gynaecologist. If the GP is reluctant to sign it because of conscientious objection, two gynaecologists independent of each other can sign the form.

2 *The pregnancy is terminated by a medical practitioner.*

The doctor should make the decision to terminate, choose the appropriate method and remain responsible for the woman's treatment throughout the abortion procedure. However, other health professionals (e.g. nurses and midwives) may carry out steps which induce the abortion (*RCN* v. *DHSS* 1981).

3 *The abortion is carried out in an NHS hospital or another approved place.*
Private clinics must be individually approved.

4 *Notification.*

Under the Act and Abortion Regulation Act 1991, the doctor who carries out the termination must notify the Chief Medical Officer using prescribed certificates. The doctor needs to supply information on the method for dating the pregnancy, the grounds for termination, the method of termination, and any complications which resulted from the procedure.

Is one of the conditions in the amended Abortion Act 1967 fulfilled?

Case 4

A 20-year-old clerk was 10 weeks pregnant for the first time. She was in a stable relationship with her boyfriend. She consulted a GP for an abortion as the pregnancy was not planned and she was concerned that the arrival of a baby would adversely affect her relationship with her boyfriend. After a thorough history and examination, the GP did not consider the risk of physical or mental harm to be excessive if the pregnancy was allowed to continue, and was not happy to sign the prescribed certificate under the Abortion Act 1967, section 1(1)(a). The woman saw another GP. Although he elicited the same history and examination findings, he agreed to sign the prescribed certificate under section 1(1)(a).

Had one of the two doctors necessarily acted illegally?

Case 5

A 24-year-old woman was 18 weeks pregnant when she was first seen in the antenatal clinic. An ultrasound scan performed at 20 weeks suggested that the baby had a congenital heart defect. A detailed scan showed simple transposition of the greater vessels, which is correctable by heart surgery. The woman requested a termination of pregnancy at 20 weeks, as she felt she could not cope with the child's surgery and post-operative period, especially as she had two other young children.

Could the doctors legally agree to the request?

In the event, the abortion was postponed due to the woman's indecisiveness. Twenty-six weeks into her pregnancy, she again requested an abortion.

Could the doctors legally agree to this request?

Case 6

A 22-year-old woman was admitted to the antenatal ward when she was 20 weeks pregnant with unusually severe pre-eclampsia. Despite bed rest, antihypertensives and sedation, her diastolic blood pressure remained high at 120 mmHg, and there were signs of eminent eclampsia. The obstetrics and gynaecology senior registrar decided that termination of pregnancy was necessary to prevent maternal fits. Unfor-tunately, there were no other independent doctors immediately available to give a second opinion.

Could a termination of pregnancy be legally performed?

Case 7

A 20-year-old woman was pregnant as a result of rape. She concealed her pregnancy from her family until the 23rd week of pregnancy. She was seen by a GP, who found her to be severely psychologically disturbed as a result of the rape and the subsequent pregnancy, and was of the opinion that continuation of the pregnancy would be extremely detrimental to her psychological health. When she was referred by her GP to the gynaecologist for termination of pregnancy, she was already 25 weeks pregnant.

Could a termination of pregnancy be legally performed?

Case 8

A 22-year-old woman was first booked into the antenatal clinic when she was 22 weeks pregnant. Her previous pregnancy resulted in the birth of a child with a syndrome asso-ciated with severe mental abnormality. The geneticist's opinion was that the prob-ability of the abnormality recurring in the present pregnancy was about 5%, and that if the child had the syndrome, the risk of severe mental handicap would be about 10%. The woman was 25 weeks pregnant when she requested a termination of pregnancy.

Could a termination of pregnancy be legally performed?

One of four conditions needs to be fulfilled. The first condition is applicable only if the pregnancy has not exceeded 24 weeks. There is no time limit for the other three conditions. The four conditions are as follows.

Section 1(1)(a): 'The social ground'

This may be applied if:

1 the pregnancy has not exceeded 24 weeks; and

2 continuing with the pregnancy would involve greater risk than if the pregnancy were terminated, or would cause injury to the physical or mental health of the pregnant woman or any existing children of her family.

Most abortions are performed under this ground. The time limit was changed from 28 weeks to 24 weeks in 1990. The time limit was chosen as a fetus above 24 weeks' gestation is considered to be capable of being born alive with current neonatal intensive care. There has been considerable debate as to whether the pregnancy should be dated from the last menstrual period (LMP) or from the implantation of the fertilized egg, which occurs 2 weeks later. It appears from the Abortion Regulation Act 1991 that the pregnancy should be dated from the LMP.

In the assessment of risk, the doctor may take into account the actual or foreseeable environment of the mother or her existing children, including social factors. This is why this condition is often called 'the social ground'. Furthermore, the risk of abortion in the first trimester is arguably less than the risk of continuing with the pregnancy, even if the pregnancy were normal.

Since the Abortion Act 1967 came into force, only one doctor has been convicted for abortion under the Offences Against the Person Act 1861. In 1973, Dr Smith was convicted after he terminated a pregnancy in a young woman in his private clinic without taking an adequate personal or social history or performing an internal examination. He was judged not to have balanced the risks involved and not to have acted in good faith. However, it would be most unlikely for a court to challenge a doctor's judgement if it was made in good faith after balancing the risks involved using information obtained from appropriate history-taking and examination.

Section 1(1)(b): To prevent grave permanent injury to the physical or mental health of the mother

The termination is necessary to prevent grave permanent injury to the physical or mental health of the pregnant woman.

An example of grave permanent injury to the mother's physical health would be severe pre-eclampsia, when termination of pregnancy may prevent serious renal or cerebral damage. Examples of preventing grave permanent injury to the mother's mental health include termination of a pregnancy resulting from rape, or when the mother already suffers from serious mental illness (e.g. schizophrenia) and is judged unable to cope with a newborn baby.

Section 1(1)(c): To reduce risk to the life of the woman

Continuing the pregnancy would involve greater risk to the life of the woman than if the pregnancy were terminated.

Examples may include eclampsia or severe uterine bleeding that were not controllable by other methods.

Section 1(1)(d): Risk of fetal abnormality or handicap

There is a substantial risk that the child, if born, would suffer from such severe physical or mental abnormalities as to be seriously handicapped.

This ground is usually used if the fetal abnormality is diagnosed after 24 weeks of gestation, as otherwise the first ('social') ground is often used instead. There is no legal definition on the degree of risk regarded as 'substantial' and the degree of handicap regarded as 'serious'. However, it is the child's handicap rather than the burden to the parents which is important.

In case 4, comparing the physical and mental risk to the mother if a termination is carried out with that in the absence of a termination is often subjective. Hence, differences in opinion amongst doctors regarding section 1(1)(a) are common. Whether the abortion is illegal rests on whether the doctor concerned has made the appropriate enquiries and balanced the risks. The courts are most unlikely to challenge the decisions made. Hence, it is likely that both doctors have acted legally.

In case 5, the abortion could be performed under section 1(1)(a) before 24 weeks. With the fetal congenital heart abnormalities, the doctors could reasonably have come to the conclusion that the risk to the mother's mental health and that of her existing children would be higher if the pregnancy continued than if the pregnancy was terminated. After 24 weeks, section 1(1)(a) could no longer be applied and section 1(1)(d) must be used instead. The risk of a transposition of a greater vessel is certain. However, it is very doubtful whether the heart abnormality would constitute serious handicap. Many doctors may consider the abnormality not serious enough. However, if doctors in good faith consider the abnormality serious enough, an abortion could be legal under section 1(1)(d).

In case 6, the mother was in imminent danger of eclampsia. Hence, the senior registrar in obstetrics and gynaecology could consider that a termination of pregnancy was immediately necessary to reduce the risk to the life of the woman (under section 1(1)(c)), or to prevent grave permanent injury to the physical health of the mother (under section 1(1)(b)). Furthermore, the Abortion Act 1967 does not require the opinion of a second doctor as the termination was immediately necessary. Hence, the doctor could proceed with the operation immediately.

In case 7, section 1(1)(a) could no longer be applied as the pregnancy was beyond 24 weeks. However, section 1(1)(b) could be applied if the doctors considered that termination of the pregnancy could prevent grave permanent injury to the mental health of the mother. The facts in this case justify the use of this section.

In case 8, section 1(1)(a) could not be applied as the pregnancy was beyond 24 weeks. The only other condition that might be applied was section 1(1)(d). The main issue was whether the risk of the occurrence of serious mental handicap to the fetus could be described as 'significant'. The risk of the child having the syndrome was 5%. If the child suffered from the syndrome, the risk of serious mental handicap was 10%. Hence, the risk of serious mental handicap was 0.5%. There is no legal definition of 'substantial' risk, and the doctor needed to make a judgement. However, many doctors may consider this level of risk not high enough to justify the application of section 1(1)(d).

Conscientious objection to abortion

Case 9

A Catholic GP was consulted by a 22-year-old woman 10 weeks into her pregnancy. She already had three young children aged 1, 2 and 4 years, and felt that both she and her children would suffer if the current pregnancy was allowed to continue. Although the GP believed that section 1(1)(a) of the Abortion Act 1967 was fulfilled, she objected to abortion morally and was most reluctant to be involved with abortion.

What should she do? Could she refuse to refer the patient to a gynaecologist?

Case 10

In case 6 above, if the senior registrar in obstetrics had a conscientious objection to abortion and no other appropriate doctors were available, could she have refused to carry out the abortion?

Case 11

If the following health professionals have moral objections to abortion, can they refuse to carry out their duties relating to abortion?
• the operating theatre staff nurse;
• the ward clerk who files the notes relating to an abortion;
• the operating theatre assistant; and
• the medical secretary who types up the consultant obstetrician's letter to the GP.

Abortion raises strong moral issues, and there are many people who have strong moral objections to it. Hence, the Abortion Act 1967 allows health professionals a right of conscientious objection, so that they would not be compelled to participate in the termination of pregnancies, even if they are under an employment contract. This only applies to health professionals who participate directly in the abortion process (e.g. nurses, doctors and operating theatre assistants) but does not include medical secretaries or clerks, or those involved in the preliminary determination of whether an abortion is justified (*Janaway* v. *Salford Area Health Authority* 1989).

An important exception to this rule is that doctors cannot refuse to treat if an abortion is necessary to save the life or to prevent grave permanent injury to the physical or mental health of a pregnant woman.

In case 9, the doctor believed that one of the conditions in the Abortion Act 1967 was satisfied, but was reluctant to participate in the abortion process. As the NHS services include abortion services, and the doctor is obliged to advise on the NHS services available, the doctor should at least refer the patient to an appropriate doctor (e.g. a gynaecologist or a fellow GP in the practice). The doctor could then avoid having to sign the prescribed form certifying that the condition for abortion was satisfied.

In case 10, the mother's life and her physical health were at risk, and a termination of pregnancy was immediately necessary. The Abortion Act 1967 does not allow doctors to refuse to treat patients under such circumstances.

In case 11, the operating theatre staff nurse and the operating theatre assistant participate directly in the abortion process, and hence have a right of conscientious objection under the Abortion Act 1967. They cannot be compelled to participate in abortion, even under a contract of employment. However, the medical secretary and the ward clerk who files the notes do not participate directly in the abortion process, and the right of conscientious objection clause does not apply to them.

Key points

1 The Offences Against the Person Act 1861 prohibits causing a miscarriage (i.e. before 24 weeks of gestation). The Infant Life (Preservation) Act 1929 prohibits the killing of a baby who is capable of being born alive (i.e. after 24 weeks of gestation).

2 The amended Abortion Act 1967 provides a defence against the Offences Against the Person Act 1861 and the Infant Life (Preservation) Act 1929 if the following criteria are fulfilled.

(a) *Medical opinion.* Two qualified medical practitioners must form an opinion in good faith that one of the conditions below is satisfied, and must sign the prescribed certificate. (If one medical practitioner has formed an opinion in good faith that a termination is immediately necessary due to (ii) or (iii) below, a second opinion is not required.)

(i) Section 1(1)(a). 'The social ground' (for pregnancy before 25 weeks). Continuance would involve greater risk than if the pregnancy were terminated of injury to the physical or mental health of the pregnant woman or to any existing children of her family.

(ii) Section 1(1)(b). To prevent grave permanent injury to the physical or mental health of the mother.

(iii) Section 1(1)(c). To reduce risk to the life of the woman.

(iv) Section 1(1)(d). Risk of fetal abnormality or handicap.

(b) *Participation of the medical practitioner.* The doctor should make the decision to terminate, choose the appropriate method and remain responsible for the woman's treatment throughout the abortion procedure.

(c) *The abortion is carried out in an NHS hospital or another approved place.*

(d) *The termination is appropriately notified.*

3 The Abortion Act 1967 allows health professionals who have conscientious objections the right not to directly participate in the abortion process. However, doctors cannot refuse to carry out an abortion if it is necessary to save the life or to prevent grave permanent injury to the physical or mental health of a pregnant woman.

References

Janaway v. *Salford Area Health Authority* [1989] AC 537, HL.
R v. *Smith* [1973] 1 WLR 1510.
RCN v. *DHSS* [1981] 1 All ER 545.

Chapter 6 – Legal issues relating to symptom relief for terminally ill patients

Managing patients for whom treatment may not confer significant benefits

In clinical practice, doctors often encounter patients whose illnesses they cannot cure. There are two particular situations in which the doctor may face a dilemma. Firstly, there is the patient who is suffering from an incurable and painful illness and who may be in so much pain that the administration of the drugs needed for the alleviation of the pain may shorten the patient's life. The doctor has to decide whether to give the drug with the intention of relieving suffering, even though it may hasten death. Alternatively, the patient might actively ask the doctor to end his or her life earlier to stop the suffering. Secondly, there are particular medical treatments which, whilst prolonging life, may not provide a net health benefit to the patient. Consideration needs to be given to withholding or withdrawing particular treatments.

Proposed treatments which may shorten the life of the patient

Case 1

A 65-year-old woman was diagnosed with carcinoma of the breast with liver metastasis and was suffering from severe pain. She implored her GP to give her an injection so that she would die quickly and peacefully.

Is it legal for the doctor to give the following treatments to achieve this aim:

1 potassium chloride injection?
2 a massive dose of diamorphine?

Case 2

A 60-year-old man was diagnosed with carcinoma of the bronchus with liver metastasis and was treated conservatively. He was treated with increasing doses of morphine. One day, he called his GP and complained of more severe pain. On examination, he also had severe respiratory difficulties. Both the doctor and the patient knew that he would soon die. On the one hand, the GP wanted to administer an intravenous injection of diamorphine to alleviate the patient's pain. On the other hand, he knew for certain that this would further depress the patient's respiratory drive and shorten his life considerably.

Could he legally administer the intravenous injection of diamorphine?

Case 3

A 45-year-old woman had been suffering from severe multiple sclerosis for some time. She was bedridden, and both the patient and her GP agreed that her quality of life was poor and the prognosis was grim. She had expressed suicidal intentions to her GP.

Over a period of weeks, she asked her GP to supply her with large doses of opiates and diazepam. A few weeks later, the GP began to suspect that she was storing up the pills so that she could commit suicide by overdose.

Would it be legal for the GP to turn a blind eye and continue to prescribe the drugs in large doses?

Murder

Under criminal law, if person A does something intending to cause person B to die, and B dies as a result, A will be guilty of murder. Hence, if a doctor administers a drug to a patient with the primary purpose of ending the patient's life and in fact does end the patient's life, he or she would be guilty of murder. The mandatory sentence would be life imprisonment.

In the case of *R* v. *Adams* 1957, Dr Adams gave an incurably ill patient high doses of opiates. He knew that the opiates would alleviate the pain, as well as shorten the life of the patient. He was acquitted of murder. The reason given was that a doctor is allowed to take all proper and necessary steps to relieve pain and suffering, even if the steps taken may incidentally shorten life. The principle that a doctor who gives pain-relieving drugs primarily to relieve pain but knowing that the drugs will also hasten death is not guilty of murder is known as the 'double effect' principle.

There are two alternative legal explanations for the 'double effect' principle. Firstly, it may be argued that the doctor does not intend to kill the patient. Secondly, it may be argued that the illness, rather than the drugs, is the cause of the patient's death. It is not clear which of these two explanations is the correct one.

In case 1, if the GP administers a potassium chloride injection, his primary purpose would clearly be to hasten death, as it would have no analgesic effect. Moreover, it is almost certain that it would cause death. Hence, the GP would be guilty of murder. This is similar to the case of *R* v. *Cox* 1992, in which Dr Cox, a consultant rheumatologist, was found guilty of the attempted murder of her patient. The patient was a lady suffering from an incurable and increasingly painful and distressing form of arthritis. The patient had previously asked the doctor not to let her suffer from severe pain, and her sons repeatedly asked the doctor to end her life. Dr Cox gave a lethal dose of potassium chloride, and the patient died soon afterwards. During the court case, the judge told the jury that, whilst the use of drugs to reduce pain and suffering will often be fully justified, notwithstanding that it will, in fact, hasten the moment of death, the use of drugs with the primary purpose of hastening the moment of death can never be lawful.

In case 1, the outcome would be less certain if the GP had administered a large dose of opiates. Strictly speaking, if the doctor's primary intention for giving the drug was to end the patient's life, then he would be guilty of murder if giving the drug, in fact, caused the patient's death. The type of drug used should not be relevant. However, it would be difficult for the Crown Prosecution Service to prove beyond reasonable doubt that the doctor's primary purpose was to hasten death and not to alleviate pain.

In case 2, if the doctor administered a dose of diamorphine, it would be clear that his intention was to alleviate pain, even though he foresaw that his actions would also hasten death. Hence, the principle of 'double effect' would apply, and he would not be found guilty of murder.

Assisting suicide

The Suicide Act 1961, section 2(1) prohibits any person to help another person to commit suicide, and the maximum sentence on conviction is 14 years' imprisonment.

In order for the doctor to be found guilty of assisting suicide in case 3, the prosecution would have to prove that the doctor intended the drugs would be used by the patient to commit suicide, that the doctor had this intent when he prescribed the drugs, and that the drugs actually helped the patient to commit suicide. In case 3, it is clear that the doctor did not intend the patient to use the drugs to commit suicide when they were prescribed. Hence, it is very unlikely that the doctor would be found guilty of assisting suicide.

The term 'euthanasia' is often used to mean intentional ending of life by artificial means of persons suffering from incurable illness. Voluntary euthanasia (i.e. a free and voluntary request from the patient) is allowed under strict regulations in some countries, such as The Netherlands. It remains completely illegal in the United Kingdom. The main argument against voluntary euthanasia is the 'slippery slope' argument—that it would be difficult to prevent involuntary euthanasia (i.e. without the patient's free and voluntary request) if voluntary euthanasia was allowed.

Withholding and withdrawing life-prolonging treatments which may not confer net benefits

In clinical medicine, there may be situations in which, although medical treatment is available to prolong a patient's life, the treatment may not bring net benefits to the patient and may be futile. Examples are premature neonates on ventilation who suffer from serious neurological deficits and patients with persistent vegetative state. If treatment has not been started, the clinician has to decide whether to withhold or to proceed with the treatment. If the treatment has already been started, the clinician has to decide whether to withdraw the treatment. Such decisions raise important legal and ethical issues, and the psychological and emotional burden on relatives of the patient and staff is heavy. There is recent guidance from the British Medical Association (BMA) (1999).

The primary purpose of medical treatment is to help the patient to maintain health, to maximize benefits and to minimize harm. Hence, medical treatment should be given only if it brings net benefits to the patient. For example, although prolonging the life of a patient usually provides benefits, it is not always the case if the quality of life would be poor, or if death would be inevitable. Many parties may be involved in the decision-making process: the patient, the relatives and the multidisciplinary health-care team.

Legally, it is important that valid consent is obtained before decisions on withholding or withdrawing treatments can be made. The general issues of consent have already been discussed in Chapter 1. The first step is to decide who can give valid consent. Consent can be divided into three categories:
• competent adults and adults with valid advance directives;
• adults who lack capacity to make decisions; and
• children and young people below the age of 18 years.

Adults

Case 4

A 50-year-old man suffered from end-stage renal and liver failure and had a very poor quality of life. He had recently suffered a myocardial infarct. The man was mentally alert and informed the physician in charge of his care that he would not like to be admitted to the coronary care unit for monitoring, and that he would not like to be resuscitated if he had a cardiac arrest. The physician could not persuade him to be admitted to the coronary care unit and observed him in the general ward. Three days later, the patient had a cardiac arrest as a complication of his myocardial infarct and the physician was urgently called.

Should the physician attempt to resuscitate him?

Case 5

A 65-year-old chronic smoker who suffered from severe chronic obstructive airway disease was admitted to the medical ward with respiratory infection and worsening respiratory failure. The patient was comatose and was in imminent danger of death unless he was artificially ventilated. There were no advance directives from the patient. The consultant in charge thought that if the patient were artificially ventilated and given intravenous antibiotics, the chance that he could be weaned off the ventilator (i.e. benefit from the treatment) was probably about 15–20%. The consultant was worried that once the patient was on the ventilator, he would not be allowed to withdraw the treatment subsequently.

Should the consultant artificially ventilate the patient? Which procedures should be followed?

Case 6

A 23-year-old man was involved in a road traffic accident. He was admitted to the intensive care unit and was ventilated. He was gradually weaned off ventilation over the next few weeks. However, he remained unarousable. A consultant neurologist found that the patient was not brain dead and was not in imminent danger of dying. However, he diagnosed a persistent vegetative state. The patient had not previously indicated how he would like to be treated if he developed this condition. His mother requested that artificial nutrition and hydration should be withdrawn to allow him to die peacefully, as continuing artificial nutrition and hydration would be futile. The clinician in charge agreed that this would be wise.

What should he do?

In the event, the patient was ventilated that night by another consultant who was on duty. During the next few days, the patient remained comatose and his blood gas did not improve. It was clear that the patient would never be able to survive without artificial ventilation, and that the treatment given was merely prolonging the patient's life without any benefits.

What should the consultant do?

Adult patients who have the required mental capacity have the final right to decide whether to accept the medical treatment offered to them. Similarly, valid advance directives (i.e. instructions given by the patient before he or she becomes mentally incompetent) refusing life-prolonging treatment have legal validity and must be followed. Hence, in case 4, the patient's instructions given 3 days earlier that he did not wish to be resuscitated if he had a cardiac arrest had legal force, provided that the patient's instructions had been given freely. Hence, the doctor must respect this instruction and should not resuscitate the patient. If he did, he could be liable for a charge of battery.

In case 5, the patient did not have full mental capacity, and there were no valid advance directives. In England and Wales, relatives of a patient cannot give legally valid consent to treatment. In such cases, the clinician in charge of the patient's care may provide treatment if it is considered necessary and in the patient's best interests. Whether the treatment is in the patient's best interests is a clinical matter. If the clinician has any doubt, he may ask for a second opinion. In this case, the consultant felt that the treatment may bring benefits to the patient, but was worried that if treatment was given, he would not be allowed to withdraw the treatment at a later date. This is a common misconception amongst clinicians. In fact, there is no legal or moral distinction between withholding or withdrawing treatment, and it is quite legitimate to start treatment and then to withdraw it if it proves ineffective.

In case 5, the patient was ventilated by another consultant, but the treatment proved to be ineffective. Withdrawal of treatment should be considered. There should be discussion with the rest of the health-care team and relatives who are close to the patient. If it is agreed that there would be no net benefits, the clinician in overall charge of the patient's care may withdraw the treatment. If the decision is seriously challenged (e.g. by the relatives), the medical defence organizations should be consulted, and review by a court should be considered.

In case 6, the patient was diagnosed as suffering from a persistent vegetative state. The dilemma is that the patient may have survived for several years if artificial nutrition and hydration were continued, although he would not be aware of his surroundings or be able to interact with other people. However, it is debatable whether artificial nutrition and hydration constitute medical treatment, and whether death caused by deliberate withdrawal of basic amenities would constitute murder. These issues have been discussed in *Airedale NHS Trust* v. *Bland* 1993. As there have been recent reports that several wrong diagnoses of persistent vegetative state have been made, a multidisciplinary team should make a thorough and appropriate assessment of the patient's condition, including the patient's potential for self-awareness and awareness of others. According to the BMA guidelines (1999), a clinical review by an independent senior clinician should be conducted. If withdrawal of artificial nutrition and hydration is considered appropriate, a court declaration that this is not illegal should be sought.

Children and young people under 18 years

Case 7

A woman who was 33 weeks pregnant was admitted to the labour ward without a previous antenatal booking. The baby was delivered with respiratory distress syndrome, and was immediately resuscitated and ventilated. The baby was then diagnosed as having Down's syndrome. The mother was distressed by the baby's future handicap and requested the paediatrician to withdraw ventilation immediately so that he would die peacefully.

What steps should the paediatrician take?

Case 8

An 8-year-old boy with end-stage cystic fibrosis was admitted to the general paediatric ward with severe respiratory failure. The paediatrician carefully explained to his mother that the child might soon die, and that artificial ventilation would not be beneficial and would certainly not be indicated. The child's mother reacted very angrily, and demanded that her child be ventilated.

What should the paediatrician do?

Case 9

A 15-year-old girl suffered from a relapse of her osteosarcoma. Metastases were found, and the prognosis was thought to be poor. The medical team offered a choice of either combined radiotherapy and chemotherapy or palliative treatment only. The clinician in charge considered that the benefits of the treatment would be minimal. The girl was sufficiently mature to understand the treatment and decided that she would not wish to have it. However, her mother insisted that she should have the treatment.

What should the paediatrician do?

Treatment of a child or young person under 18 years may proceed if legally valid consent is obtained. Generally speaking, those with parental responsibility are legally entitled to give or withhold consent to treatment. For babies or young children who are not yet sufficiently mature to understand the medical treatment, the decisions of those with parental responsibilities are usually decisive. However, if they refuse treatment and their decisions are clearly not in the child's best interests, the health-care team may apply to the courts for an order to override those decisions.

In case 7, the clinician assessed the patient clinically and decided that ventilation was in the neonate's best interests. He should discuss the likely prognosis in detail with the child's parents. Most likely, the parents would agree with the clinician, and the treatment could be continued. However, if the parents insist on withdrawing ventilation, and the clinician considers that this would not be in the baby's best interests, the clinician should seek a second opinion from another senior clinician. If the parents still refuse consent to the baby's treatment, an application can be made by the health-care team to the High Court to override the parents' decision.

In case 8, the clinician considered that ventilation would not confer net benefits on the child, but the child's mother insisted on the treatment. Although parents can give legally valid consent to treatment, they have no right to insist on treatment. Hence, the paediatrician should discuss the situation carefully and sympathetically with the parents. A second opinion from another senior clinician should be offered. However, the clinician should not feel obliged to offer the futile treatment requested by the parents.

For children who are over 16 years, or those who are sufficiently mature to understand the nature of the medical treatment, they may also give legally valid consent. If a young person accepts medical treatment, it would be legally valid. Young persons can also legally refuse treatment unless their decisions are clearly not in their own best interests. Only in extreme situations would it be justified for the health-care team to apply to the High Court to override a young person's refusal.

In case 9, the girl was clearly sufficiently mature to understand the nature of the medical treatment offered and the consequences. Her refusal of treatment was not unreasonable. Hence, her decision should be respected and treatment should not be given. Although the parents' consent to treatment is not legally valid, their decision could override the girl's refusal if the refusal is clearly not in her best interests.

Key points

Proposed treatments which may shorten the life of the patient

• If a doctor does something to the patient (e.g. giving an injection) with the primary purpose of hastening death, he or she would be liable to a charge of murder.

• If a doctor gives a treatment for the purpose of relieving symptoms (e.g. alleviating pain) but which incidentally also hastens death, this would not be illegal.

Withholding and withdrawing life-prolonging treatments which may not confer net benefits

• Treatment which does not confer net benefit to the patient can be legally and morally withheld or withdrawn.
• There is no legal or moral difference between withholding and withdrawing treatment.
• In evaluating the benefit of a treatment, its effect on both the length and the quality of life must be assessed.
• The decisions made by a mentally competent adult or an adult with a legally valid advance directive must be respected.
• If an adult is not competent to make decisions and there is no valid advance directive, the clinician in charge of the patient's care may provide treatment if it is necessary and in the best interests of the patient.
• Those with parental responsibility can give valid consent to treatment for children and young people under the age of 18 years. The views of young people aged 16 years or more or children with sufficient maturity to understand the medical treatment must be taken into account.
• If the health-care team believes that the decisions of the parents are clearly not in the child's best interests, an application may be made to the High Court to override their decisions.
• Before deciding to withhold or withdraw life-saving treatment, a multidisciplinary team must make a thorough and appropriate assessment of the patient's condition, including the patient's potential for self-awareness and awareness of others.
• Good communication with other health-care staff and the patient's relatives is essential.
• A declaration from the court must be sought before artificial nutrition or hydration is withdrawn from a patient.

References

Airedale NHS Trust v. *Bland* [1993] AC 789.
British Medical Association (1999) *Withholding and Withdrawing Life-prolonging Medical Treatment: Guidance for Decision Making.* London: BMJ Books.
R v. *Adams* [1957] Crim LR 365.
R v. *Cox* [1992] 12 BMLR 38.

Part 2
Legal Settings in which Health Professionals' Actions may be Challenged

Chapter 7 – Introduction to different legal settings in which health professionals' actions may be challenged

Introduction

The actions of health professionals can be directly or indirectly challenged via one of many legal channels:
- employer disciplinary action;
- investigation of alleged serious professional misconduct or poor performance by the professional bodies;
- NHS complaints procedures;
- medical negligence claims in the civil courts; and
- prosecution for criminal negligence.

The trends

Health professionals have been recently challenged in formal settings much more frequently than before. For example, before the 1980s, it was almost unknown for doctors to face criminal prosecution as a result of their work. However, several doctors have been charged with serious criminal offences such as manslaughter in the last few years. Patients now sue health professionals more frequently, and GPs have to pay much higher defence union subscriptions than before. The number of doctors being suspended by their managers increased four-fold between 1997 and 1998. Not only has the referral of doctors to the General Medical Council (GMC) increased, the GMC has recently introduced new procedures for assessing doctors who are thought to be performing poorly.

Unfortunately, these trends are likely to get worse, especially for medical staff, for at least two reasons. Firstly, with the recent publicity surrounding the case of the heart surgeons in Bristol who were found guilty of serious professional misconduct, the public is likely to make complaints against doctors more readily in future. Managers will also be more cautious and take action against doctors more readily. The second reason is that, under the recent NHS White Paper, all hospital managers are responsible for the quality of the health services they provide (i.e. clinical governance). One way managers can do this is by taking actions against health professionals who are thought to be performing badly.

The following case study illustrates how different procedures may be used.

Case 1

The facts

Nurse A was working as a staff nurse in a medical ward of a district hospital. The patient concerned was a 65-year-old man admitted with a mild myocardial infarct and pneumonia. He was prescribed intravenous amoxycillin together with other drugs. Nurse A was looking after the patient one evening and was administering intravenous drugs to patients. She drew up the intravenous amoxycillin in one syringe, but also drew up some potassium chloride to put in an intravenous bag for another patient. Unfortunately, she was called away by another patient. When she returned to administer the intravenous injection, she mixed up the syringes and mistakenly injected potassium chloride into the 65-year-old man. As a result, he rapidly developed dysrhythmia, suffered cardiac arrest and died.

The procedures used

The nurse manager informed the hospital managers, who suspended nurse A at once and investigated the matter fully. The coroner conducted an inquest, but adjourned the hearing as the Crown Prosecution Service was considering prosecuting nurse A. A year later, nurse A was tried in the Crown Court for manslaughter. Ten days later, she was relieved to be acquitted. The coroner then restarted the inquest, and returned a verdict of misadventure. The managers also referred nurse A to the United Kingdom Central Council for Nursing, Midwifery and Health Visiting (UKCC), who found her guilty of professional misconduct and erased her name from the register. The patient's wife sued the Hospital Trust 18 months after his death. Her claim was settled out of court for a relatively small sum.

The reasons for so many different settings

There are so many settings because each of them serves a different purpose. In some settings, the main purpose is directed against the health professional (e.g. the professional body hearing for serious professional misconduct, criminal prosecution). However, this is not the case for other settings (e.g. coroner's inquest, patient's claim for compensation, NHS complaints), even though what the health professional did may be highly relevant and vigorously challenged.

The different procedures are conducted and decided by different groups of people. They may be started off by different people. The criteria used to judge the issues are different. The consequences for the health professionals concerned are different. The differences between these settings are shown in Table 7.1.

It is therefore not surprising that more than one procedure may be used, even for a single untoward event. I have chosen a case study with particularly serious consequences to illustrate this. Apart from a few exceptions, the outcome of one procedure generally does not have direct bearing on whether another procedure will be used, or on its outcome. One exception is that any conviction in a criminal court will automatically be reported to the appropriate professional body by the police, and the facts leading to the conviction will be taken by the professional body as proven. Managers may also refer health professionals to their professional bodies or to the police after their disciplinary procedures.

Table 7.1 *A comparison of the different settings in which a health professional's actions can be challenged.*

Procedure	Who conducts it?	How is it started?	Purpose	Criteria used	Possible outcomes
Employer's disciplinary proceedings	Trust managers	Reports from patients, nurses and doctors	To protect patients	Breach of employment contract Employment law	Warning Suspension from work Dismissal from post
Professional bodies (e.g. GMC, UKCC)	Health committee Professional Conduct Committee Professional Performance Committee (GMC only)	Patients, nurses, doctors and managers	To assess fitness to practise	Guidance from the body, e.g. 'Duties of a Doctor' from GMC	Admonition Conditions attached to registration Suspension from register Erasure from register
Criminal negligence	Criminal court (jury)	Crown Prosecution Service	Punishment	Gross negligence	Absolute or conditional discharge Suspended imprisonment Imprisonment
Negligence claim	Civil court (judge)	Patients	Compensation	'Bolam test'	Financial compensation to patients
Coroner's inquest	Coroner	Upon report of death	To decide place, time and cause of death		Verdict on cause of death
NHS complaints	Stage 1: hospital managers Stage 2: independent panel	Patients, relatives	To resolve complaints To improve the service		Explanation or apologies from managers to patients

The next seven chapters will discuss some of these settings: NHS complaints procedures, professional negligence, the professional bodies and employer disciplinary actions. The role of coroners is discussed in Chapter 15.

How can we prevent this happening to us?

Although the above settings have different purposes and consequences, the ways to reduce the chance of their occurrence are similar.
- Keep up knowledge and skills.
- Recognize our limitations and ask for advice when necessary.
- Engage in meaningful communication and negotiation with patients.
- Be familiar with the policies in the hospital we are working in and follow them.
- Make accurate medical notes, especially after an untoward event.
- Join a defence organization or a trade union.

What should we do if we are threatened with these procedures?

- Try to find out which of these procedures are being used, and their purposes.
- Do not send out an angry response.
- Make some personal notes on the details leading up to the incident.
- Seek advice from the defence organization or trade union.

Chapter 8 – The NHS complaints procedure and the NHS Ombudsman

Purpose of the NHS complaints procedure

The NHS complaints procedure is a mechanism to resolve complaints if patients or relatives are dissatisfied with any NHS service or treatment. There are two purposes for this procedure:
- to resolve complaints, e.g. by explanation or apologies; and
- to improve the quality of NHS services.

Patients cannot obtain compensation from the NHS complaints procedure. They have to pursue their negligence claims through the civil courts. Although the complaints procedure occasionally results in the health authority reporting health professionals to their professional bodies, the main purpose of the procedure is not to discipline health professionals.

A national review in 1994 found significant delays in the handling of NHS complaints. Hence, a new and simplified procedure was introduced in 1996. In general, there are two stages to the new complaints procedure:
- local procedures; and
- review by independent panel.

If the complainant is dissatisfied, he or she may consider complaining to the NHS Ombudsman.

How the NHS complaints procedure works in practice

Although there are separate complaints procedures for hospitals and general practice, they are very similar. The following is a description of the general practice complaints procedure.

All general practices are required to have an in-house complaints procedure which conforms to national guidelines issued by the NHS Executive (1996). According to the guidelines, the general practices must give written information about the complaints procedure (e.g. practice complaints leaflet) to anyone who enquires, and they should publicize the procedure. Complaints should be made within 6 months of the date of the incident that caused the problem. If the patient did not discover the problem immediately after the incident, he or she should complain within 6 months of the date of discovering the problem, provided it is within 12 months of the incident.

The complaints procedure leaflet should include the following information:
- how a complaint will be dealt with;
- the purpose of the procedure;
- the anticipated timetable;
- possible outcomes of the procedure;

- the rules of confidentiality;
- the time limits for making a complaint;
- the availability of help from the local community health council;
- the availability of conciliation services through the health authority; and
- how to pursue a complaint with the health authority if the person complaining is not satisfied with stage 1 of the investigation.

Stage 1: local procedures

In each practice, there should be a person responsible for the complaints procedure. Complaints to the practice may be made verbally or in writing. When a complaint is made, the person responsible in the practice should fill out a complaint form with the complainant's details and the nature of the complaint and should give a copy of the practice complaint leaflet to the complainant.

An appointment should be made for the complainant to see the complaints administrator (usually the practice manager) to discuss the complaint in detail. The complaints administrator should keep detailed records of the meeting. The complainant should be sent an acknowledgement letter within 2 days of the interview.

The practice manager should then discuss the complaint with the staff responsible and the overseeing partner (usually the senior partner) in order to decide how to respond. The response may be a written explanation, a written apology or an offer to see the complainant again to discuss the matter further. The complainant should receive a response within 10 working days of the initial interview.

Complainants who feel unable to communicate with the practice staff directly may seek help from two other sources.

1 *Community Health Council* (CHC). It will advise anyone who wishes to make a complaint by giving practical advice on the complaints procedures, writing a formal complaint, ensuring that the complaints are followed up, and may even represent complainants in official hearings. However, it has no power to investigate the complaints.

2 *Health Authority Complaint Officer.* The Health Authority Complaint Officer may act as a mediator between the practice and the complainant and may offer conciliation services if necessary.

Stage 2: review by independent panel

Referral to convenor

If the complainant is still dissatisfied with the outcome of the stage 1 procedure, he or she can ask the health authority for an independent review. The

Health Authority Complaint Officer liaises with the convenor, who is a non-executive director of the health authority. The convenor has to decide whether or not to set up an independent review panel and reaches this decision with the help of:
• an independent lay person nominated by the Secretary of State for Health; and
• GPs based outside the health authority and nominated by local medical committees.
The convenor may then take one of the following courses:
• take no further action if everything possible has been done;
• refer the complaint back to the practice if it appears that the stage 1 procedure has not been exhausted;
• arrange conciliation if this might be helpful;
• set up an independent review panel to investigate the complaint; or
• advise the complainant of the right to approach the NHS Ombudsman.

Independent review stage

For non-clinical complaints, the independent review panel will consist of:
• an independent lay chairperson;
• the convenor (non-executive director of the health authority); and
• a second lay member.
Both lay persons are nominated by the Secretary of State for Health.
   For clinical complaints, there will be two independent clinicians to advise and make a report to the panel.
   The independent review panel will send its report to:
• the complainant;
• the practice with comments about service improvements; and
• the health authority.
The review panel does not have a disciplinary function and will not make recommendations about disciplinary actions on health professionals. However, the health authority may consider referring the matter to the relevant professional body or to the police where appropriate.

The NHS Ombudsman

The NHS Ombudsman is accountable to Parliament and is completely independent of the NHS and of Government. He is required to present an annual report to Parliament and summaries of selected investigation reports are circulated to health authorities, boards and trusts. The main purpose of the Ombudsman is to improve standards of service. Complaints may be made to the NHS Ombudsman only if the NHS complaints procedure has been followed but the complainant is still dissatisfied. The NHS Ombudsman can investigate

complaints against hospitals, community health services or general practices about the following:
- poor service;
- failure to purchase or provide a service that patients are entitled to receive; and
- maladministration—administrative failures such as avoidable delay, not following proper procedures, rudeness or discourtesy, not explaining decisions, not answering complaints fully or promptly, denial of access to information.

Since 1996, the NHS Ombudsman has also investigated clinical complaints about the care and treatment provided by health professionals or other complaints about GPs, dentists, pharmacists or opticians providing an NHS service locally.

However, the NHS Ombudsman cannot investigate:
- complaints which could be taken to court or independent tribunal services in a non-NHS hospital or nursing home, unless they are paid for by the NHS;
- complaints about local authority departments (e.g. social services) or government departments (e.g. the Department of Health); or
- the clinical judgement of a doctor or other health professional.

Procedure for complaints to the NHS Ombudsman

Patients, relatives and the next-of-kin of a deceased person may complain. Complaints to the NHS Ombudsman must be made no later than a year from the date when the complainant becomes aware of the problem, unless there has been serious delay in the NHS complaints procedure. The procedure for complaints to the NHS Ombudsman is as follows.

1 *First stage: deciding whether to investigate.* When the NHS Ombudsman receives a complaint, the first stage is to decide whether or not to investigate it, according to the criteria discussed above. He will write to the complainant about his decision and give reasons.

2 *Second stage: investigation.* If the NHS Ombudsman decides to investigate the complaint, a statement of complaint will be sent to the complainant and the NHS body involved, detailing the matters to be looked into. The NHS body will send medical records, documents and comments to the NHS Ombudsman. After studying the relevant documents, the staff of the NHS Ombudsman will then interview the complainant and other relevant witnesses. For clinical complaints, the NHS Ombudsman is advised by independent clinicians.

3 *Third stage: report.* When the NHS Ombudsman has examined all the evidence, he will then decide on one of the following courses of action:
- upheld (that is, substantiated);
- not upheld (that is, unsubstantiated); or
- not made out (where the evidence is insufficient for an 'upheld' finding) or incapable of being decided either way.

The NHS Ombudsman then sends a draft report to the NHS body involved to ensure that the facts stated in the report are correct, and to obtain an agreement to any apology or to implement any of the recommended remedial actions where appropriate. After the investigation, a copy of the final report is sent to:
• the complainant (with apologies from the NHS body if appropriate); and
• the NHS body involved (with recommendations for apologies or service improvements if appropriate).

Case 1

A 20-year-old woman was admitted to a surgical ward with abdominal pain. The surgeons could not make a positive diagnosis initially, but diagnosed appendicitis after 3 days. At the operation, the appendix was perforated and the woman remained in hospital for 10 days afterwards. The patient told her GP that she wished to make a complaint through the NHS complaints procedure so that she could receive compensation for her unnecessary pain and suffering.

What should the GP do?

Case 2

A mother telephoned her GP at midnight with a history that her 3-year-old son had developed difficulty in breathing over the night. The GP visited the patient and diagnosed viral tracheolaryngitis (croup) and gave the mother general advice on steam inhalation. The next morning, the mother saw the receptionist at the GP's practice and said that she wanted to make a formal complaint about the GP.

What should the receptionist do?

In the event, the mother saw the senior partner the next day, and explained that her son was admitted to hospital 2 hours after the GP's visit with increasing difficulty in breathing. A diagnosis of severe viral croup was made. The mother demanded to know why the child was not sent to hospital earlier.

What should the senior partner do?

Despite discussion on several occasions with the practice manager, senior partner and the GP concerned, the mother still felt unhappy and demanded an independent review.

What should the practice do?

The health authority decided to proceed with the independent review. A few weeks later, the practice received a report from the independent review panel. Although the panel did not criticize the GP's decision not to admit the child to hospital on the night of the visit, the report did criticize the GP for making inadequate notes after the visit.

How should the practice react?

Case 3

A general practice received a circular with a summary of the NHS Ombudsman's investigation of a complaint about a nearby practice. The NHS Ombudsman upheld a complaint about serious delay in arranging for a patient with abnormal cervical cytology to be seen by a gynaecologist.

How should the senior partner react to this circular?

Analysis of case histories

Case 1

The main issue here is which is the appropriate mechanism to achieve the patient's purpose. The patient stated that she wished to receive compensation for her pain and suffering. However, compensation is not awarded via the NHS complaints procedure. Rather, compensation can be pursued through the civil courts if negligence is proven. Hence, the GP should uncover the patient's motive. Often, what the patient really wants is to receive some explanation for the delay in diagnosis. If this was the case, she should be advised to see the clinicians involved or the complaints officer in the Trust. If she did not feel comfortable with approaching them, she could see the complaints officer in the health authority or the CHC. However, if her main motivation was really to seek compensation, she should be advised that this should be pursued through the civil courts and that she would succeed only if negligence was proven. She should be advised to see her solicitor about her case.

Case 2

On receiving the verbal complaint, the receptionist should give a copy of the practice complaints leaflet to the mother, and offer to make an appointment for her to see the complaints administrator of the practice (usually, but not necessarily, the practice manager).

Ideally, the senior partner should discuss the matter with the GP involved, and the GP should be given the opportunity to explain his decision not to send the child to hospital that night. If possible, the GP should explain his reasons to the mother as well. Assuming that the senior partner was the official complaints administrator of the practice, he should make notes of the discussion. An acknowledgement should be sent to the mother within 2 days of the interview. If he did not have a chance to investigate the matter before the interview, he should have discussions with the GP after the interview, and send a response to the mother within 10 working days of the interview. If they considered that the doctor's decision was right, the response would be the reasons for this. Otherwise, the response should include an apology. The mother should be informed of her right to approach the complaints officer in the health authority to request an independent review.

Immediately after the mother indicated her intention to ask the health authority to set up an independent review, the practice should collate all appropriate documentation (e.g. patient's clinical records, night visit book, doctor's rota, notes of stage 1 complaints procedure, etc.). The complaints officer would ask the practice for these documents. If necessary, the GP concerned should seek advice from the medical defence organization.

The practice should study the report carefully and review its policy on making adequate medical records. A practice meeting should be convened to agree on a policy and an audit should be performed after a few months.

Case 3

One of the main purposes of the NHS Ombudsman is to improve NHS services. This is the reason why the findings of the NHS Ombudsman are widely circulated. The practice should review its own cervical smear policy to ensure that similar problems would not occur there. If necessary, an audit could be conducted.

Key points

NHS complaints procedures serve two purposes:
1 to resolve the patient's complaints (e.g. by explanation or apology); and
2 to improve NHS services.
NHS complaints procedures do *not*:
• award compensation; or
• discipline health professionals.

General procedures

1 *Stage 1*: local procedures attempt to resolve complaints by local staff and managers; the CHC or the complaints officer of the health authority may assist.
2 *Stage 2*: independent review panel:
    (a) the convenor (a non-executive director of the health authority) decides whether an independent review panel should be set up; and
    (b) the independent review panel (consisting of lay and professional members) investigates complaints and sends reports to complainants and the NHS body investigated.
The NHS Ombudsman can only investigate if certain criteria are fulfilled, and usually investigates complaints involving maladministration. The Ombudsman's procedures are as follows:
1 decides whether to investigate;
2 conducts investigation;
3 reports to NHS body involved, and disseminates findings widely; and
4 implements findings.

> **Practical advice**
>
> Good communication with patients minimizes complaints. Prescribed communication procedures must be followed closely. If complaints arise:
> **1** they should be discussed with all staff involved;
> **2** adequate notes of the incident and complaints procedure should be made; and
> **3** parties involved should consider contacting defence organizations or trade unions.

References

Health Service Ombudsman (1996) *A Guide to the Work of the Health Service Ombudsman.* London: Office of The Health Service Commissioner.
NHS Executive (1996) *Practice-based Complaints Procedures: Guidance for General Practices.* Leeds: National Health Service Executive.

Chapter 9 – **Professional negligence**

What is professional negligence?

Read the following case histories and decide whether the doctors concerned would be found negligent.

Case 1

Dr Smith, a histopathologist, was shopping with his wife in the High Street one Saturday afternoon, when a middle-aged woman suddenly collapsed with severe shortness of breath. Dr Smith immediately attended to her. He established that she had a past history of anaphylaxis, and that she had an ampoule of adrenaline for emergency measures. An ambulance soon arrived. Unfortunately, Dr Smith had not practised clinical medicine for over a decade and did not feel confident to administer the adrenaline intramuscularly. The patient was taken to hospital but unfortunately died on arrival at the accident and emergency department.

All medical experts agreed that the patient would have had a good chance of survival if intramuscular adrenaline had been given earlier. Her husband initiated legal action against Dr Smith on behalf of the patient's estate.

Case 2

Dr Wilson, a GP, was called to visit a 3-year-old boy with a recent history of inspiratory stridor. She carefully examined the child and recorded her findings. Essentially, she found that the child was in moderate respiratory distress and diagnosed viral croup. She asked the child's mother to use steam inhalation, and to telephone for advice if the child's condition deteriorated. The child suddenly deteriorated in the evening, and his mother took him urgently to the accident and emergency department at the local hospital. Unfortunately, the child died soon after arrival. Post-mortem examination showed that the child had epiglottitis.

All the medical experts agreed that if the child had been admitted to hospital that afternoon, he would have had a good chance of being successfully treated. However, whilst some experts thought that the child should have been admitted based on the severity of symptoms recorded, other experts thought that Dr Wilson's action was reasonable.

Case 3

Dr White, a GP, saw a 65-year-old man in his surgery with a 6-month history of cough and hoarse voice. Dr White diagnosed chronic laryngitis and prescribed repeated doses of antibiotics. The symptoms persisted and Dr White reassured the patient. Four months later, the patient developed frank haematemesis, and attended the accident and emergency department. A diagnosis of advanced bronchial carcinoma was made and the patient died 3 months later.

The medical experts agreed that a 6-month history of hoarse voice should have rung alarm bells, and Dr White should certainly have investigated and referred the patient at presentation. However, they believed that even if the patient had been referred 4 months earlier, it would not have made any difference to his prognosis.

The patient's wife took action against Dr White claiming negligence through delay in diagnosis.

Case 4

Dr Pearson, a GP, saw a 30-year-old man in her surgery with a history of throat infection. Although it was clearly documented in the patient's medical records that he was allergic to penicillin, she failed to notice this and wrote a prescription of penicillin for him. The patient obtained the drug from the pharmacist, and discovered the mistake. He planned to return the next day to see Dr Pearson to obtain another prescription, but unfortunately was involved in a road traffic accident on his way to the surgery.

He took legal action against Dr Pearson for the damage caused in the accident. He claimed that if Dr Pearson had exercised more diligence, he would not have needed to return to the surgery and the accident would not have happened.

Case 5

Dr Edwards, a GP, saw a 20-year-old woman in his surgery. He made clinical diagnoses of both glandular fever and urinary tract infection. Both diagnoses were confirmed on laboratory investigations 2 days later. He prescribed trimethoprim for her urinary tract infection. Two days later, the patient telephoned Dr Bond, another partner in the practice, as Dr Edwards was on study leave. She informed Dr Bond that she had nausea whilst taking trimethoprim, and requested a change of antibiotics. However, the patient did not mention the diagnosis of glandular fever, and Dr Bond did not have the patient's records in front of him. Dr Bond asked the patient to collect a prescription of amoxycillin from the practice. The patient developed a severe rash from the amoxycillin and was very ill for over a week.

The medical experts were extremely impressed by the rapid and accurate diagnoses made by Dr Edwards. Whilst they fully understood why Dr Bond had prescribed amoxycillin, they considered that amoxycillin should never be prescribed for a patient with glandular fever. The patient took legal action against Dr Bond for negligence.

People often use the term 'professional negligence' loosely to mean bad clinical practice. However, the legal definition is much more precise. To put it simply, legal action for negligence is the patient's claim for compensation for losses caused by the professional. For a patient to succeed in a claim for professional negligence, *all* the following four elements must be proved.

1 The professional had a 'duty of care' to the patient.
2 The professional breached this duty.
3 The breach of this duty caused the patient's injury or other losses.
4 The patient's injury or other losses were reasonably foreseeable.

We shall examine each of these elements in more detail.

Duty of care

The law puts an onus on the doctor only if a professional relationship exists between the doctor and his or her patient. A duty of care exists if doctors hold themselves out as having special skills and knowledge, and patients consult them. Agreement to pay the doctor is not necessary. It is usually easy to establish that a doctor owes a patient a duty of care. Examples include a patient consulting his or her GP, a doctor in the accident and emergency department or a specialist in a hospital. However, English law does not impose an onus on a doctor to treat a stranger ('Good Samaritan' acts). Therefore, in case 1, Dr Smith had no duty of care to the patient and the patient's estate would not succeed in its claim for negligence.

Once a doctor has undertaken to treat a stranger, he or she may become liable if the treatment is improper and causes harm to the stranger. However, in case 1, Dr Smith did not undertake any treatment.

Breach of duty

A patient must show that the doctor has not fulfilled his or her duty in order to succeed in a claim for negligence. The doctor has a wide variety of duties which include making the appropriate diagnosis and giving appropriate treatment for the patient's condition and fully informing the patient about his or her status of health and any treatment proposed (see Chapter 1). However, it is well known that equally knowledgeable and experienced doctors often treat patients presenting with the same symptoms differently. Therefore, the courts have used the 'Bolam test' (*Bolam* v. *Friern* HMC 1957) to decide whether the duty of care has been breached—a doctor has not breached his or her duty if there is a 'responsible body of medical opinion' which would have acted in the same way in the same situation. Therefore, in case 2, the patient's claim for negligence would not succeed, as there are experts who considered Dr Wilson's action reasonable.

Causation

The patient must show that the doctor's mistake has caused the injury or other losses. In other words, the injuries would not have occurred if the doctor had not been at fault. In case 3, Dr White's clinical practice was certainly wrong. However, experts thought that the patient's prognosis would not have been different even if Dr White had diagnosed the condition earlier. Therefore, the patient's claim for negligence would not succeed.

The losses being reasonably foreseeable

The patient must show that the injury or other losses sustained were reasonably foreseeable when the doctor committed the mistake. In case 4, it is certainly true that the accident would not have happened if Dr Pearson had given the patient the correct antibiotics in the first place. However, Dr Pearson cannot be expected to foresee that her errors would result in a road traffic accident. Therefore, the patient's claim for negligence would not succeed.

Cases 1–4 show that bad clinical practice does not necessarily mean that the patient's claim for negligence would be successful.

Another common misconception is that if a patient's claim for negligence succeeds, the professional must be extremely incompetent and his or her clinical practice must be morally reprehensible. This is far from the truth. In case 5, most doctors would find Dr Bond's action understandable in the situation. However, all four criteria of negligence were fulfilled. In particular, Dr Bond breached his duty of care—no responsible body of medical opinion would prescribe amoxycillin with a confirmed case of glandular fever as he did. Therefore, the patient's claim for negligence would succeed.

Key points

• Bad clinical practice does not necessarily mean that the patient's claim for negligence will be successful. Doctors should inform patients of any mistakes made. However, they should not formally admit negligence without seeking legal advice from their defence unions.

• A successful claim for negligence does not necessarily mean that the health professional concerned has been extremely incompetent or morally reprehensible. It may happen to anyone.

• Negligence occurs if:
  (a) a duty of care existed between the person and the professional;
  (b) the professional breached the duty of care (no responsible body of medical opinion would have acted in the same way);
  (c) the breach caused the injury or other losses; and
  (d) the injury or other losses were reasonably foreseeable when the professional committed the mistake.

• Doctors must be extremely careful and methodical in their clinical practice to minimize the risk of medical litigation. There is no room for complacency. We shall explore each of the elements in more detail.

Does a duty of care exist between the person and the professional?

Case 6

A 60-year-old woman experienced a sudden onset of chest pain, and summoned her GP. However, the GP failed to diagnose her condition. Referral to hospital and treatment were delayed and the woman died a few hours afterwards. A close friend of the patient was informed about the death 3 hours later by the doctors in the hospital. This caused the friend much grief and sorrow for some time. The patient's friend attempted to sue the doctor for the grief she suffered as a result of the death of her friend. The doctor admitted negligence in the delayed diagnosis but denied liability for the friend's psychological harm.

Will the friend's legal action be successful?

Case 7

A 23-year-old woman was admitted to hospital in the first stage of labour. Fetal heart monitoring showed fetal distress, but this was overlooked by the midwives and obstetricians for several hours. As a result, a Caesarean section was delayed for many hours. The baby suffered severe asphyxia and died after a stormy period in the neonatal intensive care unit. The woman suffered major depression as a result of witnessing the death of her baby and required admission to a psychiatric ward for over 6 months. The hospital admitted liability for the death of the baby, but the compensation would be relatively small. The mother took legal action seeking compensation for her psychiatric illness.

Will her legal action be successful?

Case 8

At the insistence of his wife, a 30-year-old drug abuser sought advice from his doctor about his hepatitis B immune status. The GP arranged for appropriate investigations. However, he misread the laboratory report and mistakenly informed the man that he had immunity against hepatitis B. The patient's wife did not take appropriate precautions and later contracted hepatitis B. Furthermore, a prostitute also contracted the disease. Both the patient's wife and the prostitute sued the doctor for negligence.

Will they be successful?

Case 9

John was born severely mentally retarded due to two reasons—excessive alcohol intake by his mother while she was pregnant and mismanagement of umbilical cord prolapse by the midwife at his birth. John is now 18 years old.

Can he take legal action against his mother and the midwife for causing his disabilities?

As noted previously, once a health professional undertakes to treat a patient (e.g. via registration), the health professional immediately owes the patient a duty of care. However, the health professional does not have a duty of care to strangers.

Duty to third parties

Another question is whether health professionals have a duty of care to persons other than the patient.

Nervous shock

There have been many cases where, as a result of a medical mistake, a relative of the patient has suffered from nervous shock or psychological harm. The question is whether the health professional owes a duty of care to the patient's relatives. It was held in *Tredget* v. *Bexley Health Authority* 1994 that health professionals owe a duty to the relative only if the following criteria are satisfied:

1 the person is close to the patient (e.g. first-degree relatives);
2 the person was involved in the 'immediate aftermath' of the event;
3 it constituted a horrifying external event for the person;
4 the psychological harm was reasonably foreseeable as a result of the medical mistake; and
5 the person suffered from a well defined form of psychiatric illness which was more than natural sorrow or grief.

In case 6, there were several reasons why the doctor may not be legally liable for the patient's friend's psychological problems. Firstly, the person was not a relative of the patient, and the friend would have to show evidence of closeness with the patient. Secondly, the friend was informed about the death 3 hours after the event, and could not be said to have been involved in the 'immediate aftermath' of the event. Thirdly, although the death of the friend was unfortunate and sad, it could not be said to have been a horrifying event. Lastly, the friend would have to demonstrate that she suffered from a well defined form of psychiatric illness rather than normal bereavement.

By contrast, the mother in case 7 was more likely to succeed in her action against the doctor. Firstly, she clearly had a very close relationship with her newborn baby. Secondly, she was involved in the disaster at all times. Thirdly, the event could be said to have been a horrifying external event. Fourthly, her depression could have reasonably been foreseen as a result of the medical mistake. Lastly, she suffered from major depression, which is a well known psychiatric illness.

Medical advice which affects a third party

Sometimes, incorrect professional advice given to a patient may affect a third party. For example, the contacts of the patient may be affected in the treatment and control of infectious diseases. The sexual partners of the patient may be affected by contraceptive decisions. The legal question is whether the health professional is liable to these third parties.

It appears that health professionals may be liable to third parties whom they would reasonably be expected to know about at the time the advice was given (*Goodwill* v. *British Pregnancy Advisory Service* 1996). Hence, in case 8, the doctor would reasonably be expected to foresee that wrong advice given to the patient would place his wife at risk. However, he would not be expected to foresee that the prostitute would also be affected. Hence, the doctor has a duty of care to the patient's wife but not to the prostitute.

Treatment which harmed a fetus before birth

Liability for harm to the fetus is now governed by the Congenital Disabilities (Civil Liability) Act 1976, and applies to all births after July 1976. It gives a child the right to take legal action against those responsible for injuries caused before birth, either *in utero* or before conception. Furthermore, the child may also take legal action against those who, as a result of breach of their duties to the mother, caused harm to her unborn child. The child may take action at any time until the age of 21 years. However, the child cannot sue its own mother for injuries sustained before birth. The only exception is if the harm was sustained whilst the mother was driving a motor car, which the mother should have been insured against.

In case 9, John could take action against the midwife under the Congenital Disabilities (Civil Liability) Act 1976. However, he could not take action against his mother, even if his disabilities were caused by her excessive consumption of alcohol voluntarily.

The standard of care required

Against which standard would a doctor's performance be judged?

> ### Case 10
> A newly appointed senior house officer in paediatrics with no previous experience in the specialty saw a 1-year-old child in the out-patient department with recent cervical lymphadenopathy, fever, mouth ulcers, rash and peeling of skin on the palms, all suggestive of recent recovery from Kawasaki disease. However, the doctor did not suspect the diagnosis and hence did not arrange cardiological investigations. The doctor had also discussed the case briefly with the senior registrar, who did not see the child and asked the senior house officer to discharge the child from the clinic. The child died of rupture from a coronary artery aneurysm a year later. Coronary artery aneurysms are well recognized complications of the disease, and almost all senior paediatricians would arrange cardiological investigations.
>
> All experts agreed that whilst GPs or doctors who have no previous experience in paediatrics could not be expected to make the diagnosis, paediatricians would be expected to diagnose the disease and arrange appropriate investigations. Against which standard would the senior house officer be judged? Would the senior registrar be liable for negligence?

According to the Bolam test, the standard of care expected of professionals is judged by comparing those skilled in the particular speciality in question. For example, a GP would be judged against what is reasonable to expect of a GP, and a consultant surgeon would be judged against the standard expected of a consultant surgeon. Clearly, the expectation in the management of a surgical patient is higher for consultant surgeons than for GPs, although GPs may be expected to refer patients to more specialized surgeons if indications exist.

However, the experience of individual health professionals may differ significantly even if they are in the same post performing the same tasks. For example, a senior medical student may be acting as a locum for a house officer. A newly appointed senior house officer in a specialty (e.g. paediatrics or obstetrics and gynaecology) may have no experience in the specialty. A grade D staff nurse may be acting as the nurse in charge of a ward. When these health professionals who are inexperienced in their posts are sued for negligence, the question will arise as to whether they should be judged according to the standard expected of someone in the post, or the standard expected of someone with the same qualifications and experience as the health professional concerned. In a previous case, it was decided that a learner driver has the same level of care as a qualified driver (*Nettleship* v. *Weston* 1971). Hence, it is clear that health professionals would be judged according to the posts they hold, and inexperience would be no excuse.

This rule serves to protect the interests of patients, who would have no information on the experience of individual health professionals. On the other hand, this may be unfair to junior staff who are judged against a standard which is beyond their capability. However, the junior staff may avoid this unfairness by referring cases which are beyond their experience to more senior staff. If they carry out instructions given by senior staff, the senior staff would carry the responsibility (*Wilsher* v. *Essex Area Health Authority* 1986).

In case 10, the standard required of the senior house officer was the same as that of a doctor who was a paediatrician in a hospital. His inexperience was no excuse. However, as he had referred the case to the senior registrar and had carried out his instructions, the responsibility would then be on the senior registrar. The patient would be likely to succeed in negligence claims against the hospital who employed the senior registrar.

An error involving two or more professionals

Case 11

An inexperienced senior house officer in paediatrics prescribed an excessive dose of aspirin for a 3-year-old child with fever due to chickenpox. A staff nurse administered the drug to the child as prescribed without raising any queries. Unfortunately, the child developed Reye's syndrome. The experts agreed that aspirin should never have been given to the child, and that the dose was grossly excessive.

Who would be liable for the error: the senior house officer or the staff nurse?

Case 12

A GP saw an elderly gentleman with a chest infection and intended to prescribe amoxycillin 500 mg three times daily for seven days. Unfortunately, he wrote amitriptyline 500 mg three times daily by mistake. When the patient collected the prescription, he told the pharmacist that he had a chest infection, but the pharmacist dispensed amitriptyline as prescribed without raising further queries. The patient suffered serious side-effects from the drug.

Who would be responsible?

As health professionals work together in treating patients, they often rely on one another's judgement. The law allows one health professional to rely on the judgement of another as long as it is reasonable. However, they must question opinions or actions which appear to them to be wrong.

In case 11, there is no doubt that the senior house officer in paediatrics who prescribed aspirin inappropriately would be liable to a large extent. Whether the staff nurse was partially liable depends on whether the prescription of aspirin and the dose were clearly wrong. If not, the nurse would not be liable, as she could reasonably rely on the judgement of the doctor.

In case 12, the doctor who made the error in the prescription was clearly liable. However, it is likely that the pharmacist would also be partially liable. The patient had informed the pharmacist that he saw the doctor for a chest infection, but an antidepressant was prescribed. Furthermore, it should be clear that the dosage of the antidepressant was excessive. Hence, the pharmacist should have queried the prescription before dispensing it.

How do the courts decide what the required standard of care should be?

As mentioned previously, the courts have traditionally decided on the required standard of care using the Bolam test: a doctor is not guilty of negligence if he or she has acted in a way which would be accepted by a responsible body of medical opinion. In other words, the medical profession itself largely decides the required standard of proof. Although this is still generally true, the courts have, on very extreme occasions, questioned the reasonableness of the action even if it was supported by a responsible body of medical opinion (e.g. *Hucks* v. *Cole* 1960). It appears from recent case laws (e.g. *Joyce* v. *Wandsworth Health Authority* 1996) that the courts would be most unwilling to challenge opinions given by medical experts unless they are clearly unreasonable and do not stand up to analysis.

Causation

Case 13

A 24-year-old woman was admitted to hospital for a routine gynaecological operation. After the operation, the patient noticed a large burn mark on her flank which she did not have before the operation. She alleged that this was caused by the use of faulty diathermy during the operation, although she could not produce evidence that this was the case. The health professionals and the hospital denied that this was caused by the use of diathermy. However, they could not explain why the mark had occurred. Experts were unable to decide on the cause of the burn mark.

Would the patient be successful in her claim for negligence?

Case 14

A 65-year-old man was referred to a general medical department with cough and haemoptysis. The medical registrar arranged a chest X-ray, which actually showed a shadow. However, the medical registrar misinterpreted the chest X-ray and discharged the patient. The patient was re-referred to the consultant about 6 months later, when a diagnosis of bronchial carcinoma was made. The patient died 3 months later in spite of intensive treatment. The medical experts agreed that the diagnosis could have been made at first presentation. They estimated the chance of a 2-year survival from the disease was about 35% even if it had been diagnosed at the first visit.

Could the representative of the deceased patient sue for negligence?

The third criterion for negligence is that the breach of the duty of care caused the patient's injuries. As mentioned in case 3 above, the usual test is the 'but for' test. Patients need to show that they would not have sustained the injuries 'but for' the mistakes made by the health professionals. This is easy to show in some cases. Examples are where the surgeons have operated on the wrong limbs, or a death which occurs during a routine operation. However, it is sometimes difficult for a patient to prove conclusively that an injury was caused in the course of medical treatment. For example, in case 13, the exact cause of the burn mark could not be proved either by the health professionals or by the patient. Generally speaking, the patient has to prove causation in order to succeed in claiming negligence. If the cause of the injuries is unknown, the patient cannot succeed in proving negligence. However, if the nature of the injury is such that it is extremely likely to have been caused by the action of the health professionals (e.g. a median nerve palsy occurring immediately after a hand operation), causation would be assumed unless the health professionals could provide an alternative explanation. That is, the burden of proof has shifted to the health professionals. This doctrine is known as 'res ipsa loquitur' (the thing speaks for itself). In case 13, it may be possible for the patient to claim 'res ipsa loquitur'. If the health professionals were unable to provide a satisfactory alternative explanation for the burn mark, they may be held negligent.

On other occasions, one cannot be entirely certain whether the injuries would still have occurred if the health professionals had not made the mistake. For example, in case 14, the chance of the patient surviving the disease for 2 years was only 35% even if the doctor had made the diagnosis at the first visit. It was held in *Hotson* v. *East Berkshire Area Health Authority* 1987 that a negligence claim would succeed only if the patient could prove that it is more likely than not (i.e. over 50% chance) that he would not have sustained the injuries if the health professionals had not made the mistake. In case 14, since the chance was less than 50%, the patient would not succeed in claiming negligence.

Quantifying damages

Once the patient succeeds in a negligence claim, the main guiding principle in quantifying the damages to be awarded is that the patient should be compensated for what he or she has lost as a result of the medical accident. Damages are usually awarded under the following heads:

1 damages for 'pain, suffering and loss of amenity';
2 'special damages'—financial loss and expense incurred by the patient up to the time the case is settled;
3 'general damages'—damages for future financial loss or expense; and
4 interest on 1 and 2 above.

We shall examine the first three heads in some detail.

Damages for pain, suffering and loss of amenity

These are determined by a tariff based on case laws according to the injuries suffered. The exact amount awarded may vary a little depending on the characteristics of the patient (e.g. age, the possibility of future complications). However, the award for a simple knee injury may be about £3000, the loss of sight in one eye may be about £25 000, and the maximum (e.g. severe quadriplegia with mental impairment) may be about £140 000.

Special damages

These include financial loss and expenses incurred up to the time the case is settled. This may include:
- loss of earnings;
- medical expenses—even if the patient obtained private treatment; and
- nursing care or attendant expenses—these must be paid for, even if they were provided by a friend or relative.

General damages—damages for future financial loss and expense

Injuries with long-term or permanent consequences may attract huge awards, and this head constitutes the largest part of the damages in such cases. It includes the estimated:
- medical expenses for the patient's entire life;

- nursing and attendant expenses for the patient's entire life; and
- compensation for loss of earnings.

For each of the above items, the current expenses/loss of earnings (i.e. the multiplicand) are estimated. The 'multiplier' is worked out depending on the patient's age and the number of years' loss of earnings/expenses needed. As the victim may invest the compensation as soon as it is awarded, the multiplier is often less than the actual number of years expenses are needed or loss of earnings will occur. The multiplier is almost never more than 18, even if medical expenses will be needed for the rest of the patient's life.

It can be seen that the size of the damages depends not only on the nature of the injuries, but also on the characteristics of the victim (e.g. age, earnings before the injuries and the medical, nursing or attendant expenses required). The damages awarded do not bear any relationship to the seriousness of the mistake made by the health professional.

References

Bolam v. *Friern* HMC [1957] 2 All ER 118.
Goodwill v. *British Pregnancy Advisory Service* [1996] 2 All ER 161.
Hotson v. *East Berkshire Area Health Authority* [1987] 2 All ER 909.
Hucks v. *Cole* (1960) [1994] 4 Med LR 393.
Joyce v. *Wandsworth Health Authority* [1996] 7 Med LR 1.
Nettleship v. *Weston* [1971] 3 All ER 581.
Tredget v. *Bexley Health Authority* [1994] 5 Med LR 178.
Wilsher v. *Essex Area Health Authority* [1986] 3 All ER 801.

Chapter 10 – **Vicarious liabilities**

Liability of employers for employees' negligence

If an employed health professional is negligent in carrying out his or her duty and causes injuries to a patient or other person, the victim may clearly seek compensation from the health professional personally. However, provided certain conditions are fulfilled, the law also allows the victim to choose to seek compensation from the health professional's employer. On a practical level, there may be obvious advantages for the victim to choose the latter option. The employer is much more likely to be able to afford substantial claims for damages. Furthermore, the legal action may be brought many years after the event, and it may be difficult to trace the whereabouts of the health professional involved.

Importance of vicarious liability to health professionals

• Most health professionals are employed by the NHS. It is important to know whether any negligence claims against them are covered by the Crown Indemnity Scheme.
• Some health professionals (e.g. GPs) are employers. They may be liable for the negligence of their staff (e.g. their practice nurse) unless appropriate insurance is arranged.

General principles

The underlying legal reasoning for the employer's liability is that the employer, having created the situation where the employee may cause harm, should bear the responsibility for compensation. The conditions which must be fulfilled are:
1 the criteria for negligence against the employee were proved (as detailed in Chapter 9); and
2 the wrongful acts were committed 'in the course of employment'.

What constitutes 'in the course of employment'?

There are a number of situations in which it may be difficult to determine whether the wrongful acts committed were 'in the course of employment', although the case laws may provide a guide. Employees' acts are regarded as 'in the course of employment':
• if they were done for the purpose of the employer's business and were authorized by the employer;
• even if the harm was caused by the employee performing the acts in a wrongful manner (*Rose* v. *Plenty* 1976);

- even if the employers have previously prohibited the acts from being done in a wrongful manner (*Canadian Pacific Railway Co* v. *Lockhart* 1942);
- even if they were done outside the employee's working hours (*Ruddiman & Co* v. *Smith* 1989); and
- even if they were done outside the employer's premises (*Poland* v. *John Parr & Sons* 1927).

Employees' acts are not regarded as 'in the course of employment':
- if they were not done for the purpose of the employer's business (*Conway* v. *George Wimpey & Co Ltd* 1951), or the employees acted in a way that was clearly in breach of their contracts of employment (e.g. adopting a 'go slow' policy; *General Engineering Services* v. *Kingston and St Andrew Corporation* 1988); or
- if they were done in the pursuit of the employee's own personal vendetta (*Daniels* v. *Whetstone Entertainments Ltd* 1962).

Arrangements of medical negligence cover for doctors employed in the NHS (health circular HC(89)34 and HC(FP)(89)22)

Before 1 January 1990

Before 1 January 1990, health authorities protected themselves against potential claims against their medical or dental staff by requiring them to subscribe to a recognized professional defence organization. Any negligence claims by patients would then be made against the doctor or dentist personally. The medical defence organization would defend and negotiate the claims on behalf of the doctor or dentist, and would pay any compensation in the event of a successful claim.

The reasons for the change in the arrangement

Due to increasing numbers of successful medical negligence claims and the increasing size of the compensation awarded in the mid-1980s, doctors' subscriptions to the medical defence organizations tripled between 1986 and 1988. The defence organizations initiated differential subscription rates depending upon the perceived risk of successful negligence claims being made. This distorted the real earnings of doctors, and may have discouraged doctors from entering high-risk specialties such as obstetrics and gynaecology unless the subscription was re-imbursed by their employers. The new arrangements resulted after the Department of Health consulted fully with all interested parties.

After 1 January 1990 (the Crown Indemnity Scheme)

The health authorities or the NHS Trusts assumed responsibility for new and existing claims of medical negligence. Medical and dental staff were no longer required to subscribe to a medical defence organization as a condition of employment, although they were encouraged to continue to do so for work not covered by the Crown Indemnity Scheme, and for advice. Therefore, the position of doctors and dentists employed in the NHS is similar to that of other NHS employees.

Generally speaking, the Crown Indemnity Scheme covers work by doctors and dentists which is performed 'in the course of NHS employment'. The interpretation of 'in the course of employment' has already been discussed. Work which is covered by the Crown Indemnity Scheme includes:

• NHS work carried out by hospital doctors and dentists employed in the NHS 'in the course of employment';
• NHS work carried out by locum hospital doctors and dentists employed in the NHS 'in the course of employment';
• NHS work carried out by junior doctors who are working for independent hospitals as part of their training under their NHS contract;
• NHS work carried out by doctors or research workers employed by universities under their honorary NHS contracts;
• clinical assistant sessions in hospital under contractual arrangements;
• work carried out by doctors in public health medicine employed by health authorities;
• work carried out by clinical medical officers and occupational physicians employed in the NHS; and
• clinical trials carried out on NHS patients for whom the health authority is responsible.

Work which is *not* covered by the Crown Indemnity Scheme includes:

• private practice by consultants or associate specialists, even in an NHS hospital;
• work carried out by GPs and doctors in academic general practice;
• work carried out by GP registrars working in general practice;
• category 2 work (e.g. reports for insurance companies);
• work carried out by hospital doctors working for other agencies (e.g. the prison service);
• in-patients under a GP, if the hospital merely provides hotel services;
• advice and defence costs in General Medical Council (GMC) disciplinary, criminal and other legal proceedings;
• GP locum work, even if carried out by a hospital doctor; and
• 'Good Samaritan' acts.

(N.B. It is the time when the negligent acts or omissions took place, rather than the time when the patient takes legal action which is important in deciding whether Crown Indemnity applies.) Those who are not covered by the Crown Indemnity Scheme must join a medical defence organization, and the practical arrangements for handling negligence claims would be the same as before 1 January 1990.

Practical implications for the Crown Indemnity Scheme

Under the new arrangements, it is the health authorities or NHS Trusts who are being sued for the medical negligence of staff and are liable to pay for any compensations awarded by the courts. The health authorities or NHS Trusts therefore manage the defence of the case. This includes deciding whether to settle the case out of court, whether to admit liability and how to defend the claims.

Whilst this also applies to employees in other professions, some doctors have been uneasy about this sort of arrangement. Although the interests of the doctors and the NHS authorities coincide in most cases, they may conflict in some circumstances. A common scenario is that a patient receiving legal aid makes a small claim against the NHS Trust, which the doctors involved consider defensible. The NHS Trust may well prefer to settle the claim out of court if the amount involved is less than the legal costs would amount to, even if the case were successfully defended. However, the doctors may perceive that their reputation may be adversely affected if a negligence claim relating to their clinical management is settled out of court, and their private practice may suffer. Before 1990, the medical defence organizations took doctors' reputations seriously in deciding how to handle the claims, and made decisions based on the merits of the claims rather than on financial expediency. Since 1990, financial considerations have been more influential on the decisions taken by the health authorities and the NHS Trusts.

The official guidance for health authorities and NHS Trusts under the health circular HC(89)34 is that health authorities and those advising them should pay particular attention to any view expressed by the practitioners concerned and to any potentially damaging effect on the professional reputation of the practitioners concerned. They should also have clear regard to any point of principle of wider application raised by the case and the costs involved. As this is only 'guidance', the health authorities have wide discretion in the handling of the cases.

What can the practitioners do if their interests conflict with those of their employers? In practice, they can do very little. If the employers decide to settle the case (with or without admitting liability), the practitioners cannot interfere. If the claim goes to trial and the practitioners wish to have their interests separately represented, they must have the agreement of both parties (the person bringing the action and the NHS authorities) and the court. They would have to pay their own legal expenses as well as any costs incurred as a result of their being separately represented. Even if the practitioners belong to a medical defence organization, the union may not agree to pay for these costs without very good cause.

Key points

- An employer is vicariously liable for an employee's negligence if:
  (a) the criteria for negligence against the employee were proved; and
  (b) the wrongful acts were committed 'in the course of employment'.
- This is important to health professionals for two reasons:
  (a) most health professionals are employed by the NHS. It is important to know whether negligence claims against them are covered by the NHS; and
  (b) some health professionals (e.g. GPs) are employers. They are potentially liable for the negligence of their employees.
- The Crown Indemnity Scheme came into effect in 1990. This covers the majority of doctors and dentists working in the NHS.
- It is important for medical and dental staff to check whether their work is entirely covered by the scheme. Additional cover from the medical defence organizations may be required.
- Even if a medical member of staff is covered by the Crown Indemnity Scheme, it is still useful to join a medical defence organization, which is often a good source of practical advice.

References

Canadian Pacific Railway Co v. *Lockhart* [1942] AC 591.
Conway v. *George Wimpey & Co Ltd* [1951] 2 KB 266.
Daniels v. *Whetstone Entertainments Ltd* [1962] 2 Lloyd's Rep 1.
General Engineering Services v. *Kingston and St Andrew Corporation* [1988] 3 All ER 867.
Poland v. *John Parr & Sons* [1927] 1 KB 326.
Rose v. *Plenty* [1976] 1 All ER 97.
Ruddiman & Co v. *Smith* [1989] 37 WR 528.

Chapter 11 – **Product liability**

Introduction

Although the law on product liability potentially involves all health professionals, they generally lack awareness in this important area.

Drugs and physical appliances are amongst the most important tools available to health practitioners for the management and treatment of their patients. Effective drugs and appliances are seldom free of side-effects. Examples include almost all drugs, whooping cough vaccines which may rarely cause neurological problems and blood products which may rarely be contaminated by serious infectious agents. The law on product liability is concerned with whether a person who suffers harm as a result of using such a defective product can claim compensation, and from whom. This is especially relevant to health professionals. Whilst the manufacturers of the drugs or appliances may be primarily liable for damages caused by defects in their products, any persons in the chain of supply (e.g. pharmaceutical retailers, pharmacists, doctors, dentists and nurses) may potentially become liable unless suitable precautions are taken.

General principles

Before the 1970s, product liability was mainly governed by the general principles of contract law and negligence law. The protracted litigation related to the serious congenital abnormalities of babies born to mothers who took thalidomide during pregnancy prompted stricter laws for injuries caused by defective products. This led to the European Community Directive on Product Liability 1985, which was implemented in England under Part 1 of the Consumer Protection Act 1987. Whilst one of the main criteria for a successful claim for negligence is inadequate care on the part of the producer or supplier, the main criterion under the Consumer Protection Act 1987 is that the safety of the product is less than a customer could expect. Whilst a successful claim for negligence is based on the conduct of the manufacturer or supplier, a successful claim under the Act is based on the objective safety of the product (i.e. strict liability).

Victims of defective products may seek compensation under this Act, the law of negligence, the law of contract or a combination of these. The Act may prove to be more advantageous in most cases, although there are circumstances in which a person may prefer to sue for negligence. An outline comparison between the law of product liability under the Act and negligence is shown in Table 11.1.

Under the Sale of Goods Act 1979, a seller can be held liable if the goods sold do not correspond with their description or if they do not meet the quality conditions. There is no need to prove fault on the part of the seller. However, a

Table 11.1

	Consumer Protection Act	**Negligence**
Basis of claim	Defective product	Poor conduct (breach of duty)
Type of liability	Strict	Based on fault
When must the victim take legal action?	Before the earlier event of: **1** 10 years from the time the product was supplied; or **2** as in negligence	Before 3 years from the victim's 'time of knowledge' (may be a very long time from the time the product was supplied)
Who is liable?	Producer and those in the chain of supply	Producer; those in the chain of supply; licensing authorities

product liability claim under this Act is relatively rare in the health services for several reasons. Firstly, there is no contractual relationship in NHS treatment, although a claim might rarely occur relating to the supply of privately prescribed drugs, or the treatment of private patients by consultants. Secondly, it is debatable whether a health professional who administers drugs or physical appliances to a patient is supplying a product or providing a service. Thirdly, it is debatable whether medical products derived from humans, such as blood products, are regarded as goods. Liability under contract will not be discussed in detail.

Consumer Protection Act 1987

Part 1 of the Consumer Protection Act 1987 is based largely on the European Directive on Product Liability 1985, although the English version appears to impose significantly less strict responsibility on manufacturers than the European version.

The essence of the Consumer Protection Act 1987

According to sections 2(1) and 2(2) of the Act, the producer of a product shall be liable for damage if:
1 the product is defective;
2 the victim suffers loss or injuries; or
3 the damage is caused wholly or partly by the defect.
The 'producer' includes the manufacturer, 'own brander' and any person who has imported a product into the European Community on a commercial basis. In addition, any persons in the chain of supply are also liable if they have failed, on request, to identify either the 'producer' or their own supplier and the person who suffers harm cannot practically identify them.

Applying to the health services, the pharmaceutical companies, the pharmacies, the doctors, the nurses and any health professionals who help in the administration of a drug or an appliance are all in the chain of supply. It is usually impractical for patients to identify the manufacturers of drugs or medical appliances; hence the health professionals may be held liable unless they keep a record of the manufacturer and/or their own supplier.

The maximum time period before which the victim can take legal action is 10 years from the time the product was circulated. To allow time for the initiation of the legal process and to avoid liability, all suppliers must keep records for at least 11 years.

What are 'products' under the Consumer Protection Act 1987?

Most marketed pharmaceutical products and medical appliances are included, although it is debatable whether human blood products and human organs are. However, manufacturers are not liable for medicinal products that are used before they are marketed. Hence, if doctors or other health professionals administer such products to patients, they may be liable for any damage caused.

What are 'defective products' under the Consumer Protection Act 1987?

A product is deemed defective if 'its safety is not such as persons generally are entitled to expect'. All the circumstances shall be taken into account, including the purposes for which and the manner in which the product has been marketed. Hence, the criterion for judging safety is an objective standard rather than the producer's fault.

Like negligence, the safety of the product is judged by the standard expected at the time the product was supplied by the producer.

Possible defences

Although liability under the Act is 'strict', there are two defences which are particularly relevant to health care.

1 *The defect did not exist in the product at the relevant time* (sections 4(1)(d) and 4(2)). For example, if the side-effects of a drug are caused by deterioration resulting from a pharmacist's inadequate compliance with the manufacturer's storage instructions, the manufacturers may escape liability and the pharmacist becomes liable.

2 *The 'development risks' defence* (section 4(1)(e)). It is a defence if the state of knowledge at the relevant time was not such that a producer of the kind of products *might* be expected to have discovered the defect. This considerably weakens the 'strictness' of the liability. In deciding whether a manufacturer might be expected to have discovered the defect, the court may take into account various factors such as financial and scientific constraints.

Product liability under the law of negligence

The general principles of negligence have been discussed in Chapter 9. For a victim to claim negligence against a person or organization, the following must be proved:
1 that the person or organization owes the victim a duty of care;
2 that the duty of care was breached (the standard of care was below that reasonably expected);
3 that the victim suffered harm; and
4 that the harm was caused by a breach of the duty of care.

Who owes a duty of care?

Negligence was first applied to the issue of manufacturer's liability for defective products in the famous 'snail in the ginger bottle' case (*Donoghue* v. *Stevenson* 1932). In this case, the manufacturer was held to have a duty to take reasonable care to the ultimate consumer. Since then, negligence has been applied more widely to product liability. Besides the manufacturer and all those in the chain of supply, the Licensing Authority may also owe a duty of care to victims.

What is a reasonable standard of care?

Whether the care shown by the manufacturer was adequate is assessed by the state of technical and scientific knowledge at the time. The adherence to industry standards and guidelines produced by the Licensing Authority or the Code of Practice of the Pharmaceutical Industry is an important, though not necessarily decisive, consideration.

Manufacturers may be held to be negligent in a number of ways:
• manufacturing faults, e.g. drugs containing impurities or of incorrect strength;
• design faults, e.g. risks caused by poor design of a hip prosthesis or intraocular lens; and
• poor marketing standards: failure to warn consumers about potential risks in promotional material. It should be noted, however, that duty may be discharged by the 'learned intermediary' rule—by alerting health professionals as responsible intermediaries.

If the potential risks of a marketed product are known after it has been put into circulation, the manufacturers have a duty to warn previous users and prescribing health professionals, to issue public warnings or to recall products in circulation as may be appropriate. Hence, manufacturers need stringent procedures for monitoring adverse effects and administrating product recall. Doctors and other health professionals need to keep a good record of the manufacturer and the batch number of the drugs or appliances prescribed to patients, and to have a good system for identifying which patients have received the defective products.

Is the harm caused by the defect in the product?

A defence available to the manufacturers which is of particular interest to doctors and other health professionals is the intermediate examination defence. If a product is so obviously defective that the doctor or pharmacist who supplies the product to the patient should be reasonably expected to detect it, the responsibility may be shifted to the doctor or pharmacist involved. This highlights how important it is for all health professionals to inspect any drugs or appliances supplied to a patient for any obvious defects.

Key points

- Product liability laws are legislation designed to protect consumers.
- All producers and those in the chains of supply of products may be liable.
- Whereas negligence is based on fault, strict liability is imposed for producers of products and those in the chains of supply.
- All health professionals who administer drugs or medical appliances are in the chain of supply of such products.
- Practical steps for health professionals to minimize the risks of product liability include:
    (a) following the manufacturer's instructions literally and carefully;
    (b) documenting how the instructions have been followed; and
    (c) documenting the manufacturer and the batch number of any drugs or appliances administered to patients. These records should be kept for a minimum of 11 years.

Reference

Donoghue v. *Stevenson* [1932] AC 562.

Chapter 12 – **The professional bodies**

Introduction

It is important to the public that people working in professions such as law, accountancy and medicine are competent. Legislation exists which requires the establishment of professional bodies to maintain the standards of professionals. For example, outside health care, all accountants and lawyers are regulated by professional bodies. There are also many such professional bodies regulating health professionals. Examples are:
- the General Medical Council (GMC)—for doctors;
- the United Kingdom Central Council for Nursing, Midwifery and Health Visiting (UKCC)—for nurses, midwives and health visitors;
- the General Dental Council—for dentists;
- the General Osteopathic Council—for osteopaths;
- the General Chiropractic Council—for chiropractors;
- the General Optical Council—for opticians; and
- the Council of the Pharmaceutical Society of Great Britain—for pharmacists.

The health professions have been mainly self-regulated; traditionally, the professional bodies have been mainly run by the professionals themselves. They attempt to maintain high standards in several ways:
- keeping an up-to-date register of qualified members;
- admitting members only if they meet the basic educational and training requirements;
- removing members who become unfit to practise;
- promoting high standards of education within the profession; and
- promoting good professional practice.

The professional bodies primarily serve to protect the public from incompetent professionals, but historically have also served to give professions their status.

In recent years, the effectiveness of professional self-regulation has been seriously questioned. Professional bodies (especially the GMC) have been put under pressure to regulate their members more tightly under the threat of direct regulation by the Government. For example, the GMC established the performance procedures in 1996 by which it may deal with doctors whose professional performance appears to be seriously deficient. The Bristol heart incident in 1998 (when many young children died after being operated on by paediatric cardiac surgeons) has further challenged the efficacy of professional self-regulation. After the GMC erased the names of two of the three doctors from its register, the Secretary of State for Health announced a public inquiry and claimed that all three doctors should have been struck off the register. There was a report by a senior paediatrician appointed to the public inquiry committee, who was removed from the enquiry committee for unconvincing reasons (Smith 1998). These events raised concerns amongst health professionals that the era of professionally led professional regulation would give way to externally led professional regulation.

A frequent criticism of the professional bodies is that they do not resolve the grievances of those who complain against practitioners. The complainant is not party to the disciplinary procedures and may not even appear during the hearing. This is because the main concern of the professional body in these proceedings is to decide whether the practitioner should be allowed to continue to work in the profession. It has no authority to award compensation to complainants.

This chapter will concentrate on two professional bodies: the GMC and the UKCC. The UKCC regulates by far the largest professional group. The effectiveness of the procedures of the GMC is probably more hotly debated than those of any other health professional body. The procedures of the General Dental Council are broadly similar to those of the GMC.

The General Medical Council

There are 104 members of the GMC. Most members are doctors who are elected and other doctors are appointed by medical schools or medical royal colleges. About a quarter of the members are lay (non-medical) people who represent the public.

The basic purposes of the GMC are to protect patients and to guide doctors. The functions of the GMC include:
• keeping an up-to-date register of all qualified doctors;
• promoting high standards of medical education (e.g. by accrediting medical schools and issuing guidance on undergraduate and postgraduate medical education);
• promoting good medical practice (e.g. by issuing guidance such as 'Good Medical Practice' to all doctors); and
• taking action over doctors who may be unfit to practise.
We shall concentrate mostly on the last function: taking action over doctors whose fitness to practise is in doubt.

Procedures for handling complaints to the GMC

Complaints can be divided into three types:
1 professional misconduct issues;
2 professional performance issues; and
3 health issues.

Professional misconduct issues

The GMC may receive complaints about doctors from several sources: patients, NHS authorities, other employers of doctors and the police. At all stages, the criteria which the GMC use to judge the doctor's conduct are those in the booklet 'Good Medical Practice', which is published by the Council.

Screener stage

When the Council receives a complaint about a doctor, it will first decide whether the matter complained of is serious enough to question the doctor's registration. This is decided by a medically qualified 'screener'. The screener will examine for evidence suggesting serious professional misconduct or seriously deficient professional performance. If the screener decides that no action needs to be taken, the case will be referred to a non-medical member of the Council. If the non-medical member also agrees, the case will end. Otherwise, it will proceed to the Preliminary Proceedings Committee stage.

Preliminary Proceedings Committee

If the screener decides to proceed with the case, it will be referred to a seven-member Committee (consisting of five medical and two non-medical members) of the GMC. The Committee meets in private and considers all the evidence relating to the case. It may then decide to take any one of the following actions:
• no action;
• to send a letter of advice or warning;
• to refer the case to health procedures; or
• to refer the case to the Professional Conduct Committee for a public hearing.
Rarely, if the matter is serious, the Preliminary Proceedings Committee may suspend the doctor's registration for up to 6 months. The doctor will then be invited to attend the meeting and have a legal representative.

Professional Conduct Committee

If the case is referred to be heard by the Professional Conduct Committee, formal charges will be drafted by lawyers for the GMC. A hearing will be arranged in the GMC's office in London. The public hearing will follow formal legal procedures as in a court. Witnesses may be called by both the Council and the doctor, and may be cross-examined. Both the Council and the doctor may be represented by lawyers, and the Committee is advised by a senior lawyer on points of law.

After hearing the evidence, the Committee will decide on two questions: whether the doctor had behaved as charged, and if so, whether this amounted to serious professional misconduct. The standard of proof is the criminal standard: to prove beyond reasonable doubt.

If the Committee decides that the doctor was guilty of serious professional misconduct, it can take one of the following actions:
• to warn the doctor and close the case;
• to place conditions on the registration for up to 3 years (e.g. to limit the

specialties in which the doctor may work, to work only under supervision, not to prescribe certain types of drugs, etc.);
• to suspend the doctor's registration for up to a year; or
• to erase the doctor's name from the register.

If the doctor's name is removed from the register, the doctor can make an application for the Council to restore his or her name to the register after 10 months. The application will be considered by the Professional Conduct Committee again in a public hearing.

Appeal

If the Committee decides to impose conditions, to suspend the registration or to erase the doctor's name from the register, the doctor has 28 days to appeal to the Judicial Committee of the Privy Council. The appeal can only be on points of law.

Professional performance issues

The performance procedures were introduced in 1996 to give the GMC power to deal with doctors whose professional performance appears to be seriously deficient. This covers situations where the doctors, though not guilty of serious professional misconduct, repeatedly or persistently fail to meet the professional standards appropriate to the work they are doing.

The professional performance procedures bear a resemblance to the professional conduct procedures. However, the performance procedures are usually conducted in private and the reports of the procedures are not published.

Screener stage

The screener stage is the same as for complaints of professional misconduct above. The screener may refer the case to be dealt with by the performance, conduct or health procedures as appropriate.

Assessment Referral Committee

The screener may invite the doctor to be assessed. If the doctor does not agree, the case will be referred to the Assessment Referral Committee for consideration. If the Committee decides that the doctor should be assessed, it can order the doctor to be assessed. The doctor and the complainant both have a right to appear before the Assessment Referral Committee and to be legally represented. The meetings of the Assessment Referral Committee are not open to the public.

Performance assessment

If the doctor is to be assessed, another GMC member will be appointed as the case co-ordinator. The assessment panel will consist of two specialists and a lay person. One specialist will be from the specialty the doctor is working in and the other specialist is selected to reflect the subspecialty and the circumstances of practice.

There are different assessment protocols for different specialties, and they have largely been developed by the relevant royal colleges. Generally speaking, there are three stages.

• *Stage 1*: the assessors visit the doctor at his or her place of work to review records and discuss cases with the doctor concerned, interview the doctor and colleagues.

• *Stage 2*: the doctor may be asked to do standard tests to assess professional knowledge and skills.

• *Stage 3*: the doctor may be observed in his or her routine work.

The assessment panel will produce a report and the doctor who is under assessment will have a chance to comment on it. The case co-ordinator may then choose one of three options:

1 to find that the doctor's performance is not a cause for serious concern and to take no further action;

2 to find that there are serious deficiencies in the doctor's performance and to require the doctor to take action to deal with them (e.g. to undergo counselling or training). Restrictions may be placed on the doctor's work in the meantime. The doctor will be required to make the necessary improvement by the time of the reassessment; and

3 to find that the deficiencies in the doctor's performance are so serious that the case is referred to the Committee on Professional Performance.

Committee on Professional Performance

Doctors may be referred to the Committee on Professional Performance by the case co-ordinators either because the performance deficiencies were very serious, or because the doctor did not co-operate in the assessment process.

The Committee on Professional Performance again usually consists of five medical members and two non-medical members of the GMC. The hearing is usually held in the Council's office in London. Formal legal procedures are followed as in the Professional Conduct Committee's hearings, but the hearings are not open to the public.

Again, the Committee may receive advice on points of law from a senior lawyer. In addition, it may receive expert advice from one or more independent specialist advisors.

The power of the Committee on Professional Performance and the appeal procedures are similar to those for the Professional Conduct Committee.

Health procedures

The health procedures are used for doctors who have a serious health problem into which they themselves have little insight. Common health problems include drug or alcohol addiction and mental illness. These often put patients at risk. There are significant differences between the health procedures and the conduct/performance procedures. The main purpose of the health procedures is to protect patients whilst the doctor is supervised and treated by senior doctors with expertise in the field.

Health screeners
The health screener is usually a psychiatrist. The health screener decides whether the doctor concerned should be invited to be examined by medical examiners (consultant psychiatrists) appointed by the GMC.

Medical examination
The doctor will be asked to be examined by at least two medical examiners. They will then send reports to the health screener on the doctor's state of health and fitness to practise, make recommendations on any necessary treatment, and on any need to restrict the doctor's work while he or she is receiving treatment (e.g. to practise only under supervision).

The health screener will then make one of the following decisions:
• to close the case if the examiners report that the doctor is fit to practise;
• to ask the doctor concerned to accept the recommendations for treatment and to agree to any restrictions on work; or
• to refer the case to the Health Committee if the doctor concerned refuses to be medically examined, to accept recommendations for medical treatment or to limit the medical work carried out.

The Health Committee
Doctors may be referred to the Health Committee by the health screener, or by the Conduct/Performance Committees if they believe that a doctor's illness may be the underlying cause for the original complaint.

The Health Committee consists of seven medical and two non-medical members of the GMC. Again, formal legal procedures are followed. Apart from legal advisors, the Committee is advised by two experts: a psychiatrist and a specialist who is working in the same area as the doctor.

The power of the Committee and the appeal procedures are similar to those for the Professional Conduct Committee.

Future development: revalidation of registration

The GMC aims to introduce revalidation for all doctors in the United Kingdom by 2002. All doctors will have to submit evidence to the GMC that they are practising in accordance with clearly defined guidelines. The standards against which doctors will be judged in decisions relating to the revalidation are still being developed, but they will not be confined to clinical competencies. Communication skills, professional values, professional relationships and record keeping are also likely to be included. If there are initial doubts about a doctor's suitability for revalidation, further assessments will be conducted by assessors. In parallel to this process, the Chief Medical Officer has also proposed a compulsory annual local appraisal process for all doctors, supported by external peer review process. The information gathered in the appraisal process would provide a core of information for GMC validation. The final decision about revalidation rests with the GMC.

The introduction of revalidation of all doctors is undoubtedly partly triggered by the well publicized cases relating to services delivered by the paediatric cardiac surgical team in Bristol which resulted in two doctors being struck off the register by the GMC. These events have severely damaged public confidence in the medical profession. A public enquiry is still ongoing. It is hoped that the revalidation procedures will restore public confidence in doctors.

The United Kingdom Central Council for Nursing, Midwifery and Health Visiting

The UKCC is the statutory regulatory body for the largest health professional group, and regulates the nursing (adult, paediatric, mental health, learning disabilities and community nursing), midwifery and health visiting professions.

The UKCC is similar to the GMC in many respects. The UKCC consists of 60 members (40 elected and 20 appointed by the Secretary of State for Health). The elected members represent all three professions and all the countries in the United Kingdom. However, unlike the GMC, there are separate bodies (National Boards for Nursing, Midwifery and Health Visiting) to oversee the education of nurses. The main functions of the UKCC are:
• to maintain a register of qualified nurses, midwives and health visitors;
• to set standards for nursing, midwifery and health visiting education, practice and conduct;
• to provide advice for nurses, midwives and health visitors on professional standards; and
• to consider allegations of misconduct or unfitness to practise due to ill health. We shall concentrate on the misconduct procedures. The health procedures are similar to those of the GMC.

Unlike the GMC, the UKCC currently has no professional performance procedures. The two UKCC procedures deal with allegations of professional misconduct and allegations of unfitness to practise due to ill health. However, whilst the GMC Professional Conduct Committee can only act if it finds serious professional misconduct, the UKCC Professional Conduct Committee may act if it finds professional misconduct. This is loosely defined as 'conduct unworthy of a nurse, midwife or health visitor.' Hence, it is sometimes possible for the UKCC to deal with what are really performance problems via the professional conduct procedures.

The UKCC professional conduct procedures

Screening by case officers

The UKCC receives complaints about a nurse, midwife or health visitor from various sources: a patient, a carer, another nurse or health professional, NHS Trust managers or other employers. The complaint must be submitted in writing.

The complaints are initially screened and investigated by case officers of the UKCC, who may gather information and evidence from witnesses. The case officers will decide whether there is a case to be answered and whether the allegations might lead to the health professional's name being removed from the register if they are substantiated. If so, the case is referred to the Preliminary Proceedings Committee (PPC). The health professional complained of will be notified of the allegations.

The Preliminary Proceedings Committee

The PPC consists of Council members, practitioners and consumer representatives. The meeting is held in private. The purpose of the PPC is to ensure that only those cases which might lead to a finding of professional misconduct are referred to the Professional Conduct Committee (PCC).

The PPC can take one of the following actions:
• close the case;
• refer the case to the professional screeners for the Health Committee;
• issue a formal caution on future conduct; or
• refer the case to a formal hearing of the PCC.

Rarely, the PPC may suspend the practitioner's registration pending further investigations.

The Professional Conduct Committee

If the PPC refers the case to the PCC, a full public hearing will be held. The practitioner may choose to be represented by a lawyer or by an officer from his or her professional organization or trade union. The hearing is conducted according to formal legal rules.

In addition to Council members, practitioners and lay people, the PCC also has a legal assessor to advise on points of law. In order to find the practitioner guilty of professional misconduct, the Committee has to decide on two questions:
1 if the allegations are true; and
2 if they are true, whether they amount to professional misconduct.
The standard of proof is the criminal standard of 'beyond reasonable doubt'.

If the practitioner is found guilty of professional misconduct, the PCC can take one of the following actions:
• close the case;

- issue a caution;
- remove the name of the practitioner from the UKCC register for a specific period of time; and
- remove the name of the practitioner from the UKCC register indefinitely.

Practical advice to doctors involved in one of these procedures

If you receive notification from your professional body that one of the procedures is being used against you, you should:
- find out which procedure is being used against you;
- read the allegations against you;
- refresh your memory of the relevant incident from the health records;
- make personal notes on the details leading up to the incident;
- avoid sending out angry responses; and
- seek advice from your professional organization (e.g. medical defence organization, trade union).

They are able to offer legal advice on the procedures and to represent you in the proceedings if necessary.

Case histories

Case 1

You are the senior partner in a general practice. You have received informal complaints from patients that one of your junior partners smelt of alcohol during his home visits over the last few months. You also noticed that he had been late for work on most mornings. Two weeks ago, you noticed that he prescribed amoxycillin to a patient who was known to be allergic to amoxycillin. Other partners in the practice suspect that he has an alcohol problem and advised him to seek expert advice. However, he vigorously denied that he had a problem. On the one hand, you feel that you should not report your own colleague to the GMC. On the other hand, you feel that if you do not do so, the patients in the practice would be put at risk.

What should you do?

Case 2

You are a single-handed GP. One day, you receive a letter from the GMC informing you that you are being investigated for serious professional misconduct. A complaint was received from a patient of yours alleging that you failed to visit her 2-year-old daughter 4 months previously, and she died as a result. You are asked to give comments about the complaint. You do not remember any details about the visit request.

What should you do?

After examining the evidence, the Preliminary Proceedings Committee decides to refer your case for a formal hearing by the Professional Conduct Committee.

What should you do?

Case 3

You are a GP trainer. One day, your GP registrar informs you confidentially that he has recently been convicted of possessing a small amount of cocaine for his own personal use. Although the magistrate dealt with him leniently by giving him a conditional discharge, he was worried that his name would be erased from the medical register.

How would you advise him?

Case 4

You work as a junior partner in a three-doctor general practice. Over the previous year, you and the other junior partner have noticed that the senior partner has become gradually out of date with his medical knowledge, and that his clinical work has deteriorated. He has no interest in continuing medical education and his clinical records are illegible. On one occasion, he prescribed a beta-blocking agent to a patient who had asthma. Fortunately, the patient did not suffer serious harm, and there have been no complaints from the patients. The senior partner does not appear to suffer from poor physical or mental health. You and your partner have discussed these problems with him informally, but he did not appear concerned.

What can you do?

Analysis of case histories

Case 1

Alcohol problems are relatively common amongst doctors. In this case, the problem appeared to affect the doctor's professional work. The senior partner should first try to resolve the matter informally by discussing the problem with the doctor. The doctor should be advised to see his GP to be referred to appropriate specialist help. Alternatively, he should be advised to contact one of the following organizations for informal advice:

• the Sick Doctors' Trust national helpline for addicted physicians (Tel: 01252 345 163) which provides 24-hour advice and an intervention service; or

• the National Counselling Service for Sick Doctors (Tel: 0171 935 5982).

The senior partner could also seek help from local medical committees for assistance.

However, if the doctor concerned refused to seek advice, the senior partner should carefully assess the risk to his patients. Under current GMC guidance, all doctors are obliged to inform the GMC about sick colleagues if they believe the risks to patients are real and significant. The senior partner should inform the GMC by contacting the Council's fitness to practise division, which may give informal advice and guidance about invoking the GMC's health procedures.

Case 2

The GP should try to find out exactly what happened. The patient's medical record, the visit book and the night visit book should be carefully studied. If on-call duty was shared with other practices, the duty doctor roster should be obtained to ascertain who was on call that night. A list of patients who consulted the practice that day should be obtained to assess the workload of that particular day. Other staff (e.g. receptionists, the practice nurse) may remember vital details.

All relevant information should be documented as far as possible. In view of the serious nature of the complaint, the GP should seriously consider contacting the medical defence organization for assistance in drafting a reply to the GMC. The reply should begin by expressing sympathy for the death of the child, and should provide a factual account of what happened that day: whether the practice received a request for a visit, whether the doctor attended and what the doctor did. Angry responses should be avoided.

When the Preliminary Proceedings Committee decides to refer the case to the Professional Conduct Committee, the medical defence organization must be contacted. All relevant documents and other evidence must be carefully collated in preparation for the hearing.

Case 3

The GP trainer should advise the GP registrar that the police routinely report convictions of any doctors to the GMC. The GMC would regard the facts leading to the conviction as proven.

From the information given, it is likely that the screener would refer the case to the Health Committee rather than to the Professional Conduct Committee. The GP registrar may need to undergo a medical examination by a medical examiner appointed by the GMC. The GMC has power to attach conditions to the doctor's registration. It also has power to erase the doctor's name from the register, although it is unlikely to do so from the facts given.

Case 4

The doctor's problem appeared to be chronic poor performance due to inadequate medical knowledge and skills. The other partners in the practice would need to decide whether the lack of skills and knowledge were sufficiently serious to put patients at risk.

They should first try to resolve the matter by discussing it informally with the doctor, if necessary with the help of the local medical committee.

Before 1997, the GMC had no power to deal with doctors whose professional work was generally seriously deficient, but who had not been involved in an incident which constituted serious professional misconduct. However, the GMC can now deal with such doctors using the professional performance procedures.

Whether to invoke such procedures would be a difficult decision for the junior partners. They would have to balance the risks to the patients and the harmful effects on relationships within the practice very carefully.

Key points

• Professional bodies exist by Laws of Parliament to maintain standards of health professionals and to protect the public.
• Currently, most health professions are self-regulated. However, the effectiveness of self-regulation has recently been challenged by the public.
• The role of professional bodies includes:
  (a) keeping a register of qualified members: admitting only those with appropriate qualifications and removing those who are unfit to practise; and
  (b) issuing appropriate guidance on professional conduct and professional education.
• Professional bodies do *not*:
  (a) award compensation; or
  (b) provide explanations or apologies to patients.
• A health professional may be unfit to practise because of:
  (a) poor health;
  (b) professional misconduct; or
  (c) poor professional performance.
• Practical ways to minimize the risks of being accused of being unfit to practise include:
  (a) maintaining good communication with patients and colleagues;
  (b) keeping up to date with medical knowledge and skills;
  (c) being familiar with the guidance from the professional bodies;
  (d) making and keeping adequate clinical records;
  (e) registering with a GP and seeking professional advice for illnesses; and
  (f) joining a defence organization or a relevant trade union.

References

Buckley G (1999) Revalidation is the answer. *British Medical Journal* **319**; 1145–6.
Department of Health (1999) *Supporting doctors, protecting patients. A consultation paper on preventing, recognising and dealing with poor clinical performance of doctors in England.* London: Department of Health.
Smith R (1998) Regulation of doctors and the Bristol inquiry. *British Medical Journal* **317**; 1539–40.
Southgate L, Pringle M (1999) Revalidation in the United Kingdom: general principles based on experience in general practice. *British Medical Journal* **319**; 1180–3.

Chapter 13 – Relationship between employers and employees

Introduction

Some doctors are employed, whilst others are self-employed. In general, most hospital doctors, general practice trainees and assistant GPs are employees. On the other hand, most principal GPs are self-employed. They act as employers and may employ assistant or locum GPs, practice nurses and administrative staff. Most nurses are employees.

The same employer–employee relationship applies whether doctors act as employers or employees.

Differences between employees and the self-employed

Some important legal differences between employees (e.g. hospital doctors) and the self-employed (e.g. GP principals) are as follows.
- The National Insurance payments are different.
- Employees pay income tax under Schedule E in the pay as you earn (PAYE) scheme. Self-employed people pay income tax under Schedule D.
- The health and safety protection given to employees is more extensive than that given to self-employed people.
- The employer is vicariously liable for negligence committed by the employee. Hence, NHS Trusts are generally financially responsible for negligence committed by health professionals in the course of their duty, including doctors (under the Crown Indemnity Scheme). GP principals are financially responsible for negligence actions taken against them. Hence, they must take out a medical defence insurance.

Legal issues which often arise in the employment relationship

The following three issues are particularly important for doctors, both as employers and employees, and this chapter will focus on them in particular.
1 Unlawful discrimination (in the selection process, treatment of current employees and in dismissal and redundancy).
2 Terms and conditions of employment.
3 Disciplinary matters (including dismissal).

Unlawful discrimination

General principles

Unlawful discrimination is an important employment issue. Not only is unlawful discrimination an important issue in selection, it is also an important issue in all employment processes—from the selection process (job advertisement, handling of enquiries from potential applicants, shortlisting the interview stages) to treatment of employees, disciplinary matters and redundancy.

Two main forms of unlawful discrimination were introduced in the mid-1970s: sex discrimination (under the Sex Discrimination Act 1975) and race discrimination (under the Race Relations Act 1976). The law relating to these two forms of discrimination is rather similar, and they will be discussed together. A third form of unlawful discrimination, disability discrimination, was introduced under the Disability Discrimination Act 1995, and will be implemented in stages. Legislation on age discrimination is being contemplated.

Sex and race discrimination

Read the following case histories. Consider whether there has been unlawful discrimination, and if so, which type of discrimination.

Case 1

A male doctor who had just completed his house officer posts was shortlisted for a senior house officer post in obstetrics and gynaecology. Three other doctors were also shortlisted and interviewed, two males and one female. After the interview, the female applicant was offered the post. The chairman explained to the unsuccessful applicants afterwards that the committee preferred female trainees as all the patients in the specialty are women.

Case 2

A female Registered Mental Nurse B applied for a staff nurse post in an acute psychiatric ward. The nurse visited the personnel department to make enquiries about the post and was informed by a personnel officer that the committee would prefer candidates who were over 5 feet 7 inches tall, in order to manage violent patients effectively. However, nurse B was just under 5 feet 4 inches. She applied for the post, but was not shortlisted for interview without specific reasons. A male Registered Mental Nurse who was 6 feet tall was appointed.

Case 3

An article in one of the medical journals analysed all applications to medical schools in the previous 2 years. It found that ethnic minority applicants had a significantly lower chance of being offered a place than white applicants in several medical schools. These results were corrected for the actual A-level results, although data on teachers' prediction of A-level and GCSE results, which are usually used in making decisions regarding admissions, were not available in the analysis. An Asian school leaver applied to one such medical school. He met the basic conditions for acceptance but was not offered a place. His actual A-level results were above the average of those who were admitted to the medical school that year.

Case 4

Dr D applied for the post of a senior house officer in general medicine, with on-call duty one in every four weekends. He was about to be offered the post, when he informed the committee that, due to his religious beliefs, he would not be able to work on Saturdays. The committee offered the post to another candidate.

Under sex and race discrimination, the following three main types of discrimination are possible.

1 *Direct discrimination .*

This occurs when a person of one sex (or ethnic group or married persons) is treated less favourably than a person of another sex (or ethnic group), or the sex (or ethnic group or single persons) of that person is the reason for the unfavourable treatment.

2 *Indirect discrimination.*

This occurs when:

(a) the employer applies a condition or requirement to the applicants;

(b) the proportion of persons from one sex (or racial group, or married persons) who can satisfy that condition or requirement is considerably less than that of the other sex (or racial group, or single persons);

(c) this is to the detriment of the applicant who complains because he or she cannot satisfy the condition or requirement; and

(d) the employer cannot show that the condition or requirement is justified.

An important difference between direct and indirect discrimination is that, whilst the employer may justify indirect discrimination with reasons, direct discrimination is not capable of justification. (N.B. It is not unlawful to discriminate against single persons in favour of married persons.)

3 *Victimization.*

It is also unlawful to victimize a person because he or she has attempted to take legal action or to give information or evidence alleging discrimination.

What remedies are available?

Individuals

Claims of sex or racial discrimination may be submitted to an industrial tribunal within 3 months, although the period may be extended if it is fair to do so. If the complaint is upheld, the tribunal may order compensation to be paid to the complainant. If the behaviour of the employer was judged to be outrageous, large exemplary damages may be awarded. If appropriate, the tribunal may also order the employer to take action to reduce the adverse effect of the alleged behaviour.

Commission

The Equal Opportunities Commission (for sexual discrimination) or the Commission for Racial Equality (for racial discrimination) can conduct a formal investigation.

Comments on the case histories

Case 1

The male doctor was clearly treated less favourably than the female applicant and his sex was clearly a reason for this. Hence, there appeared to be a case of direct sexual discrimination. Direct discrimination is not generally capable of justification, unless sex is regarded as a genuine occupational qualification for the post. Posts in which sex or race may be regarded as genuine occupational qualifications are very rare. Hence, the male doctor could claim unlawful direct sexual discrimination according to the facts.

Case 2

In this case, the reason that Nurse B was not appointed to the post was probably because of her short stature, and not directly due to her sex. Hence, the employer's behaviour did not constitute direct sexual discrimination.

The next question is whether the employer's behaviour fulfilled the criteria for indirect sexual discrimination.

The employer appeared to have applied a condition of a height of more than 5 feet 7 inches. It can easily be shown statistically that a higher proportion of men satisfy this criterion than women. The application of this criterion appears to have been detrimental to the applicant, as she was not offered the post. Hence, there was indirect sexual discrimination. This would be unlawful if the employer could not justify applying the condition. Whether the criterion is justified would depend on several factors, such as the existing staffing level, the general level of violence on the ward, the relative importance of physique and training in managing violence, etc.

Another issue is whether Nurse B could rely on the remark made by a personnel officer in pursuance of her discrimination claim. Past case laws suggested that she could, especially if the personnel officer appeared to have acted as a 'first filter' for selection (*Brennan* v. *Dewhurst Ltd* 1984).

Case 3

The relationship between the applicant and the medical school is not an employer–employee relationship. Nevertheless, the sex and race discrimination laws discussed above similarly apply. There was no direct evidence that the reason the Asian student was not offered a place was because of his racial origins.

However, the results of the journal article suggest that the chance of obtaining an offer was lower for an ethnic minority applicant than for a white applicant. If the results are valid, one might intuitively reason that the medical school was either directly discriminating against ethnic minority applicants or was applying conditions that a considerably smaller proportion of ethnic minority students than white students could satisfy (indirect discrimination). However, the law requires the person who brings an action to prove either direct or indirect discrimination (or both). To demonstrate indirect discrimination, the person bringing the action would need to state a criterion which is more easily satisfied by white applicants than by applicants from ethnic minorities. For example, the Asian student may choose prediction of A-level results as a criterion, but he would have to show that teachers generally underestimate the performance of students from ethnic minorities. This shows that proving indirect discrimination is often very difficult.

Furthermore, statistics are often not clear-cut. For example, the medical schools may argue that they also rely on GCSE results and personal references in making decisions, and analyses of such data are very difficult to find.

Case 4

As a result of his religious beliefs, Dr D was unable to work on Saturdays and he was not offered the post. Dr D clearly could not claim direct racial discrimination for two reasons. Firstly, racial grounds in the Race Relations Act 1976 include colour, race, nationality, ethnic and national origins. However, the Act does not cover religious groups. Secondly, even if religious groups were covered by the Act, there are no obligations on employers to alter the job description to cater for applicants' religious beliefs.

Key points in relation to sex and race discrimination

• Unlawful sex and race discrimination may occur in all employment issues— the selection process, the treatment of current employees, disciplinary matters, dismissal and redundancy.
• Discrimination against either males or females is unlawful.
• Discrimination against married persons in favour of single persons is unlawful.
• Discrimination on the basis of colour, race, nationality or ethnic origins is unlawful.
• Discrimination may be direct or indirect. Indirect discrimination can be justified with good reasons. Direct discrimination cannot.
• Victimization of those who take actions, give evidence or provide information in these procedures is unlawful.

Disability discrimination

The Disability Discrimination Act 1995 aims to eliminate discrimination against disabled persons, and the Act is brought into force in stages. Until December 2000, it does not apply to an employer who employs fewer than 20 people, although this number will be reviewed around December 2000.

Case 1

A 30-year-old woman, Mrs E, applied for an out-patient receptionist post in a hospital. She was permanently wheelchair bound due to paralysis of both legs after a road traffic accident. She had no disability other than her mobility. The receptionist post mainly involved administrative work when patients attended the out-patient clinic, which Mrs E was well capable of doing. However, occasionally when the Medical Records Department was short-staffed, receptionists would have to shelve the medical notes in the Medical Records Department. Mrs E found this duty difficult. Furthermore, the door in the reception area which separated the patients and the staff would have had to be widened to allow wheelchair access.

Is it lawful for the NHS Trust to refuse to offer Mrs E the position because:

1 she would be unable to shelve medical notes?; or

2 adjustments would have to be made to the door?

Who are disabled persons under the Disability Discrimination Act 1995?

The Secretary of State for Employment has issued detailed guidance on the matters to be taken into account in determining questions relating to the definition of disability. There is also a Code of Practice for the elimination of discrimination in the field of employment against disabled persons or persons who have had a disability.

Under sections 1–2 of the Act, a person is disabled if:
- he or she has a physical or mental impairment;
- the impairment has a substantial and long-term adverse effect on the person's ability to carry out normal day-to-day activities*; and
- the impairment has lasted for at least 12 months, or would reasonably be expected to last for that period or for the rest of the person's life. However, if the impairment ceases to have a significant impact on a person's ability to carry out day-to-day activities but it is likely to recur, it can still be treated as having that effect.

The fact that a person is disabled under some other classification (e.g. he or she is claiming disability living allowance) does not automatically mean that the person is classified as disabled under this Act.

* A physical impairment must affect a person's mobility, manual dexterity, physical co-ordination, ability to carry objects, speech, hearing, vision, memory and ability to concentrate or to learn in order to satisfy this criterion. A mental impairment must form a well recognized clinical illness.

What is discrimination under the Disability Discrimination Act 1995?

An employer discriminates against a disabled person if, without good justification, he or she:

1 treats a disabled person less favourably than a person who is not disabled; or

2 fails to make adjustments to arrangements (in relation to employment, promotion, transfer or training) or physical features of premises to minimize any substantial disadvantage suffered by the disabled person (section 6).

To determine whether it would be reasonable for an employer to make adjustments, multiple factors are taken into account, such as:

• the effect the adjustment would have on the disabled person;

• the financial and other costs involved compared with a comparable person without the disability; and

• the availability to the employer of financial and other assistance to make the necessary adjustments.

However, other than the duty outlined under section 6, employers are not required to treat disabled persons more favourably than other employees.

What remedies are available?

The individual can make complaints to an industrial tribunal. If upheld, the tribunal can:

1 make a declaration to this effect;

2 award compensation; or

3 recommend that the employer takes action to minimize the discriminatory effect.

Comments on the case history

The issues to address are as follows.

1 *Did the Disability Discrimination Act 1995 apply to the employer?* As the Trust certainly employed more than 20 employees, it did apply.

2 *Was Mrs E disabled under the Disability Discrimination Act 1995?* As her mobility was permanently affected, her physical impairment constitutes disability under the Act.

3 *Could the Trust refuse to offer Mrs E the post because of her inability to shelve medical notes?* The Act does not allow the Trust to treat Mrs E more unfavourably than other persons because of her disability without good justification. This is true both in the selection process and in the treatment of her after her appointment.

In general, treatment is justified if it is the result of applying a condition under which the amount of a person's pay is wholly or partly dependent on that person's performance, if the condition is applied to all of the other employer's employees who are doing similar jobs and if it is not directed specifically at the disability.

In the case of Mrs E, it would only be lawful to refuse to offer her the post due to her inability to shelve the notes if this formed a significant part of the duty of a receptionist. Circumstances differ between hospitals, but it would appear that shelving notes would not form a significant part of the job in Mrs E's case. Hence, it would be unlawful for the Trust to refuse her the post for this reason.

4 *Could the Trust refuse to offer Mrs E the post as adjustments needed to be made to the entrance, which would be unnecessary if another person was appointed?* Under section 6 of the Act, the Trust was obliged to make adjustments, unless there was good justification why this could not be done. The cost of making the adjustment for an NHS employer would be small and the effect to Mrs E would be significant. Hence, it would appear that it would be unlawful for the Trust to refuse to offer Mrs E the post for this reason.

Key points in relation to disability discrimination

• The Disability Discrimination Act 1995 applies to employers with 20 or more employees.
• The concept of indirect discrimination does not apply.
• Employers have a duty to make reasonable adjustments so that the disabled person would not suffer substantial disadvantage.

Good practice in the selection process for employers

Advertisements

• Vacancies for most health professionals (e.g. doctors, nurses) should be advertised in a national professional journal (e.g. *British Medical Journal, Nursing Times*). Practice clerical and administrative posts may be advertised in local newspapers.
Advertisements should:
• clearly specify the nature of the post and essential and desirable criteria for the post;
• state how the person specification may be obtained;
• state that the employer is an Equal Opportunity Employer (if appropriate); and
• avoid clauses which may be interpreted as directly or indirectly discriminatory.

Application forms

• If application forms are used, applicants need not disclose their sex, nationality or ethnic origin (unless a separate form is used for monitoring purposes).

Shortlisting

- Apply the criteria specified in the advertisement and person specification.
- Make brief notes of the reasons for those not shortlisted.

Interviewing

- Ask questions which are relevant to the criteria stated in the person specification.
- Avoid questions which are specific to a particular sex, race or nationality without good justification.
- Avoid direct questions on future plans for children.
- It is permissible to ask about a disability: how it may affect job performance and what adjustments may need to be made.
- Make brief notes on reasons for rejection.

Terms of employment

Case 1

Several consultant anaesthetist posts within an NHS Trust remained vacant, partly due to a national shortage of qualified anaesthetists. Repeated advertisements for the vacancies failed to attract suitable candidates. As a result, elective operations had to be cancelled. The managers in the Trust were prepared to attract suitable candidates by paying higher salaries and relocation expenses than were nationally agreed.

Was this legal?

Case 2

A full-time receptionist at a general practice under a permanent contract left her job. The general practice principals decided to replace her with two part-time receptionists under short-term 1-year contracts.

Was this legal?

Case 3

A consultant surgeon was informed by the Trust managers that the Trust Board had decided that (a) although the registrars and senior registrars previously saw a proportion of new cases referred, the consultant must now personally see all new cases referred by GPs; and (b) no two consultant surgeons should be away on annual or study leave at the same time. Furthermore, the consultant annual leave entitlement would be reduced from the normal 6 weeks to 5 weeks. The consultant felt that these changes were not in his contract of employment, and therefore could not be legally imposed on him without his consent.

Was he right?

The employer–employee relationship is essentially that of an agreement between two parties. Generally speaking, the employer agrees to pay the employee and take certain precautions to ensure the employee's health and safety, whilst the employee agrees to perform tasks at a certain time and in a certain place. Exactly what has been agreed is usually set out in the contract of employment. We often hear people talk of 'terms and conditions of employment'. In fact, terms and conditions are different. Terms are part of the agreement between the employer and the employee, and may include such issues as salary, duties involved and annual leave entitlement. Changes should be agreed by both parties. On the other hand, conditions are unilateral instructions from the employer to the employee and include such issues as how salaries are paid, how the work is performed, when the annual leave can be taken, etc. For example, a house officer's duties including caring for in-patients are a term, whereas which equipment should be used in taking blood is dictated by the Trust's policy, and is a condition. A senior house officer being entitled to 5 weeks' annual leave is a term, whereas the policy that no more than one senior house officer in a clinical firm may be on leave at the same time is a condition.

The agreed terms of employment are central in determining legal issues arising from employment. If the employee is in breach of contract, the employer may discipline the employee. If the employer is in breach of contract, the employee may take legal action for compensation or to require the employer to fulfil the terms of the contract. If the employee is dismissed, a claim of unfair dismissal can be made.

Although the terms of employment are generally set out in the employment contract, there are two exceptions. Firstly, the courts and tribunals may infer terms from the contract when they are not expressly stated in the employment contract. For example, it is implied that the employer will treat the employee with respect and trust, and will give the employee reasonable time off work to deal with a domestic emergency (*Warner* v. *Barbers Stores* 1978) and will not falsely accuse an employee of theft (*Robinson* v. *Crompton Parkinson Ltd* 1978). There is also an implied duty of not disclosing confidential information about the employee to third parties, and an implied duty to ensure the employee's health and safety at work. Similarly, an employee is expected to use appropriate skill and care, to be competent in the work he or she is employed to do and to obey reasonable orders.

Secondly, a national collective agreement (e.g. General Whitley Council regulations) may be made between an employee's association (e.g. the Department of Health) on the one hand and the trade union (e.g. British Medical Association) on the other. The terms negotiated in the collective agreement may be incorporated into the employment contract. This may be explicitly stated in the employment contract, or may be implied. Hence, the terms of employment for an individual employee may be changed by a revised collective agreement, if the changes are accepted collectively by the trade union.

Comments on the case histories

Case 1

The Review Body on Doctors' and Dentists' Remuneration usually gives recommendations to the Government on the appropriate level for doctors' salaries each year, and doctors' salaries are decided by the Government nationally. However, as an individual employer, an NHS Trust can lawfully change the recommendations if this departure from national recommendations is explicitly stated in the individual employment contract and is agreed by both employers and employees. However, it may not be wise to do so on a practical level. The professional organizations (e.g. the British Medical Association) may object to such practice. Furthermore, if all NHS Trusts adopted this strategy, it would lead to a spiralling of doctors' salaries without any improvement in the recruitment situation in the country as a whole.

Case 2

There are no national terms of employment for general practice receptionists. Hence, the general practice principals can legally employ two part-time receptionists under fixed-term contracts, as long as that is agreed by both parties.

Case 3

The change in Trust policy that all new referrals from GPs should be seen by the consultant is a change to the way he performs his work. Hence, it is a change in condition, which can be unilaterally imposed by the employer.

Similarly, the policy that no two consultants could be away at the same time is a change in the condition of employment, which could be imposed unilaterally. However, the reduction of the length of annual leave entitlement is a change in explicit employment terms which could not be imposed on the consultant without his consent.

General principles

• Employment terms are usually stated explicitly in the employment contract, although they can be implied from the circumstances or incorporated as part of a collective agreement.
• Terms can usually be changed with the agreement of both parties. Conditions can be imposed unilaterally by the employer.

Practical notes on written particulars of the contract of employment

According to section 1 of the Employment Rights Act 1996, the employer must give the employee a written statement within 2 months of the start of employment with the following details.

1 Basic information:
  (a) the names of the employer and the employee;
  (b) the title of the employee's job;
  (c) the place of work and the address of the employer;
  (d) the date on which employment began;
  (e) the date on which the employee's period of continuous employment began; and
  (f) if employment is not expected to be permanent, the period for which it is expected to run. For fixed-term contracts, the date when it is to end.
2 Remuneration:
  (a) the scale or rate of remuneration; and
  (b) the intervals at which remuneration is paid.
3 Hours of work, leave entitlement and pension scheme:
  (a) hours of work;
  (b) holidays and holiday pay;
  (c) sickness leave and pay entitlement; and
  (d) pension scheme.
4 Length of notice:
  (a) length of notice employee is required to give to end the contract; and
  (b) length of notice employee is entitled to receive to end the contract.
5 Collective agreements:
  any collective agreements which directly affect the terms of employment.
6 Grievance and disciplinary matters:
  (a) disciplinary procedures; and
  (b) grievance procedures.

Disciplinary powers of employers

Case 1

Staff nurse F was employed under a permanent contract by an NHS Trust. One day, two elderly in-patients complained to the managers that nurse F had hit them whilst they were on the ward. The managers immediately suspended staff nurse F with full pay and fully investigated the matter, including taking full statements from the patients. They also reported the matter to the police. The Crown Prosecution Service (CPS) decided that there was insufficient evidence to charge the nurse. A full disciplinary hearing was held in accordance with the Trust's disciplinary procedure. The Trust found the nurse guilty of gross misconduct and dismissed her from her post, as well as informing the United Kingdom Central Council for Nursing, Midwifery and Health Visiting (UKCC).

The staff nurse argued that the fact that the CPS decided not to prosecute her showed that the Trust managers were wrong to dismiss her.

Was she right?

Case 2

Complaints were made against a consultant physician by five patients about the quality of medical treatment. The consultant was suspended on full pay and an enquiry was conducted by the Trust managers with the assistance of two independent consultant assessors. They found that the consultant was hard-working and conscientious, and there was no evidence of misconduct. One independent consultant felt that the standard of the management of the five patients was just acceptable, although the other felt that it was somewhat below what would be expected of a consultant physician. An assessment of his general competence was marginal. The Trust managers were anxious to protect the public from unnecessary risk and did not wish to reinstate the consultant.

What are the options for the managers and the consultant?

Case 3

A full-time receptionist was employed by a general practice under a 3-year fixed-term employment contract. At the end of the 3 years, the general practice principals did not renew the contract and appointed another full-time receptionist in her place.

Can the receptionist claim that she was unfairly dismissed?

Case 4

A ward sister was employed under a permanent contract and had been working in an NHS Trust for over 3 years. She did not get on well with her new manager. She felt that the manager often criticized her work unreasonably, and undermined her authority in front of more junior nursing staff and other health professionals. She had previously reported these events to senior managers. One evening, the manager walked into the ward and accused her of incompetence and dishonesty in front of all the junior nursing staff, medical staff and patients. In anger, the ward sister left her job that evening of her own accord.

What legal claim, if any, did she have on her employer?

Generally speaking, an employer may discipline an employee if the employee has broken a term in the employment contract. The employer has the responsibility of drawing up the disciplinary procedure, and must give a note to each employee specifying any disciplinary rules which are applicable to them, and any appeal procedure. The actual rules which an employee is expected to observe may be found either in the disciplinary procedure itself, or in the staff rules or policy, or a combination of both. Rules may be divided into two types:

1 general rules which define types of conduct which cannot be tolerated in an employer–employee relationship; and

2 specific rules which apply specifically to the particular employer–employee relationship.

Examples of general rules governing conduct which may lead to disciplinary actions include theft from the employer or from fellow employees, serious neglect of duty, dangerous practice, etc. Specific rules depend on the nature of the post. For example, a 20-minute delay in answering an emergency call may lead to disciplinary action for a junior doctor, but not for a receptionist.

The disciplinary powers are usually detailed in the disciplinary documents. However, in general, they may include:

- warnings;
- reprimands;
- demotion;
- transfer;
- alternative employment;
- suspension (with or without pay); and
- dismissal.

When a disciplinary matter is suspected, the managers must conduct the investigation and disciplinary hearings fairly. Otherwise, the employee may successfully appeal against any disciplinary actions taken. Until recently, disciplinary procedures relating to personal conduct for all NHS staff were governed by section 40 of the General Whitley Council Conditions of Service. Most NHS Trusts have now drafted their own procedures following the Code of Practice on Disciplinary Practice and Procedures in Employment (1977), which was developed by the Advisory, Conciliation and Arbitration Service (ACAS), although employers are not legally obliged to follow this Code. The supervisor or manager should first investigate and find out the facts quickly, taking statements from any available witnesses. In serious cases (e.g. when patients may be at risk), the employee may be suspended with pay. The employee involved should be interviewed and given the chance to state his or her case, and should be advised of his or her rights under the disciplinary procedures, including the right to be accompanied (e.g. assistance from a trade union). The disciplinary procedures should be followed in detail. Records should be kept, including details of any breach of disciplinary rules, the action taken, the reasons for the action and whether an appeal was lodged.

The action the employer takes depends on the seriousness of the matter. For minor offences, the employee might be given a formal oral or written warning, detailing the nature of the offence and the likely consequences of further offences. Further misconduct might attract a final written warning and the statement that any recurrence would lead to suspension or dismissal. The final step might be disciplinary suspension without pay or dismissal, depending on the nature of the misconduct.

Summary dismissal is a strong measure, and can be justified only under the most exceptional circumstances. These may include gross misconduct, dishonesty and gross neglect of duty.

The employee may challenge the employer's decision in the following situations using appeal procedures and the industrial tribunal. The employee may succeed if:

1 the employer did not follow a fair procedure. The employee will succeed even if the unfairness of the procedure did not alter the outcome of the disciplinary procedure (*Polkey* v. *A. E. Dayton Services Ltd* 1988).

In assessing whether the procedure was fair, the following points are important:
• the employee should be informed of the nature of the charge against him or her in sufficient detail to enable him or her to prepare the case;
• the employee should be given an opportunity to state his or her case, no matter what the circumstances are;
• he or she should be permitted the right to have a trade union representative or another employee to speak on his or her behalf;
• he or she should be informed of the right of appeal to a higher level of management or to an independent arbitrator;
2 the employer's decision must be reasonable under the circumstances. For the decision to be reasonable:
• the employer must have informed the employee previously that the conduct concerned would attract the disciplinary action given;
• the rules should be clear and readily understandable;
• the employer must be able to justify any differences in treatment between different employees; and
• the decision itself must be considered reasonable by the tribunal.

Procedures for disciplining hospital doctors

The disciplinary procedures for hospital doctors have been updated by the health circular HC(90)9. It appears that NHS Trusts are obliged to follow it, as it is an implied term of the employment contract that the employer will give regard to such a national circular (Raymond 1992). HC(90)9 distinguishes between professional misconduct (i.e. the performance or behaviour of doctors, such as rudeness or violence) and professional incompetence (i.e. inadequacy of the performance of doctors in exercising their skills and professional judgement, such as poor standards of diagnosis and treatment).

The procedures for professional misconduct are broadly similar to the ACAS guidelines. There are two procedures for professional incompetence. With less serious allegations, the medical director first informs the doctor about the complaints. He or she then asks the Joint Consultants' Committee to nominate at least two independent assessors from outside the district to investigate the matter in private and in the absence of the doctor involved, and to produce a report for the medical director. The medical director will then decide what action to take, and the doctor may appeal against his or her decision. With serious allegations, the NHS Trust usually suspends the doctor on full pay pending a full enquiry hearing. For consultants, there is a right to appeal to the Secretary of State for dismissal, though not for summary dismissal.

New proposals for NHS employers to deal with poorly performing doctors

The Chief Medical Officer proposes a comprehensive system enabling NHS employers to deal with poorly performing doctors. The proposal is under consultation at the time of writing.

Compulsory periodic appraisal

It is proposed that all doctors (including junior doctors, hospital consultants and GPs) would be compelled to undergo regular appraisal and review of their performance and personal development plans by their employers. This process will be supported by an external peer-reviewed process. It is proposed that the appraisal process should have a series of core strands including work performance, participation in local clinical governance, adherence to General Medical Council (GMC) guidelines and continued professional development including teaching and research.

New proposed mechanisms to resolve problems of poor clinical performance

The existing disciplinary procedures governing professional misconduct and incompetence were perceived as ineffective and its abolition was proposed. The main perceived problems for the existing system are the need for long periods of suspension and time-consuming investigations.

Step 1: Local service action

Under the new proposals for dealing with problems of poor clinical performance, the first step is for the employer (represented by the Medical Director and Human Resources Director) to decide which of the following categories the problems fall into.

1 *Concerns about clinical performance or professional conduct.* This would lead to an Assessment and Support Centre referral.

2 *Misconduct of a personal nature* (e.g. criminal offence, harassment at work). This would be dealt with under the employer's internal disciplinary procedure, as is currently the case.

3 *Failure to fulfil contractual commitments* (e.g. not turning up for work commitments). This would be dealt with under the employer's internal disciplinary procedure under the new proposals.

4 *Serious clinical dysfunction.* In serious cases, direct referral to the GMC should be considered.

Step 2: Assessment and support centres

Under the new proposals, Assessment and Support Centres run jointly by the NHS and the medical profession will be established. In each centre, there will be a Medical Director, a Board of Governors, and a lay Chairman. Information may be gathered from records, documentation, clinical audits, interviews with the doctor, and site visits. The Centre would provide a diagnosis of the problem, a full written assessment of its nature and seriousness, and recommendations for actions. The assessment will be sent to both the doctor and the Trust (for hospital doctors) or health authority (for GPs).

The Centre may recommend monitoring according to specified criteria, a period of re-education and retraining followed by reassessment, re-skilling in another area of medical practice followed by reassessment, referral to formal GMC procedures, referral for medical treatment (similar to the current sick doctor procedures), or referral to the employer with a report that the problem is serious and intractable.

Step 3: Further action
The Trust (for hospital doctors) or health authority (for GPs) will implement the recommendations with the doctor. The doctor may appeal through the NHS Trust or health authority mechanisms. If the employer decides to terminate the doctor's employment because there is no prospect of remedial action, the doctor may appeal to the industrial tribunal. However, it is proposed to remove the existing right of appeal to the Secretary of State.

Dismissal and unfair dismissal

What is dismissal?

Dismissal can take place in three main ways (there is also a fourth: when a woman intends to return to work after maternity leave, but is not permitted to do so by her employer).

1 *Employer termination.* Dismissal occurs when the employment is terminated by the employer with or without notice. This is so even if the employee invites this course of action. The employer inviting the employee to resign also constitutes dismissal.

2 *Expiry of a fixed-term contract.* If the employee is employed for a fixed term, a dismissal occurs if the contract is not renewed after its expiry.

3 *Constructive dismissal.* If the employer's conduct amounts to a significant breach of the employment contract and the employee leaves the employment with or without notice, constructive dismissal is said to have occurred.

What is unfair dismissal?

A number of questions should be addressed to determine whether dismissal has been unfair.

1 *Is the employee eligible to claim unfair dismissal?* In order to claim unfair dismissal, the employee must have had continuous employment with the same employer for more than 2 years. However, this period may be reduced when the case of *R. v Secretary of State for Employment* ex p Seymour-Smith and Perez, HL, 13 March 1997 is heard by the European Court of Justice.

2 *Has there been dismissal?* See 'What is dismissal?' above.

3 *Has the dismissal been unfair?* For contracts terminated by the employer, whether the dismissal was unfair depends on the fairness of the procedures used and the reasonableness of the situation. In cases where a fixed-term contract is not renewed, it depends on whether there is a genuine need for an employee to have a fixed-term contract, or whether it is only a means of dressing up an ordinary job to deprive employees of their rights. For constructive dismissal, it depends on whether the employer's conduct was so unreasonable that it amounted to a significant breach of the contract.

Comments on the case histories

Case 1

The allegations that the nurse had hit elderly patients were so serious that the managers were fully justified in suspending her on full pay. The managers were correct to report the incident to the police, and the disciplinary processes appeared to be full and fair.

There are several differences in the criteria that the CPS use to assess whether to proceed with prosecution and those used by managers to decide on disciplinary matters. Firstly, second-hand and hearsay evidence would be inadmissible in a criminal court and would be disregarded by the CPS, whereas it may be proper for managers to rely on it. Secondly, to secure a conviction in a criminal court, the offence must be proved to a very high standard, that of 'beyond reasonable doubt', whereas managers in a disciplinary hearing need not prove that the offence took place, but must merely act reasonably in coming to a decision. Therefore, the decision of the CPS not to pursue the prosecution is entirely compatible with the managers' decision on disciplinary matters.

Case 2

The disciplinary procedures for hospital doctors under the health circular HC(90)9 should be applied.

The managers were justified in suspending the consultant physician pending investigations, in order to protect other patients. In many complaints which call into question the competence of doctors, opinions may differ amongst experts. In this case, there was no suggestion of misconduct, and the reports of the independent assessors did not appear to give sufficient evidence of incompetence to justify dismissal. However, the managers did not have confidence in reinstating the doctor. In the past, hospital managers suspended such consultants on full pay for a prolonged period of time, on some occasions for more than 10 years. This was wasteful of NHS resources as well as being damaging to the doctors' careers, especially as the skills of the doctor would decline further if he or she was not engaged in active practice. The 1990 health circular now lays down strict time limits for suspension on full pay. The options in this case were to negotiate with the consultant regarding further training or to transfer him to another post, although the doctor could not be compelled to comply under the law of employment.

However, since the introduction of professional performance review procedures by the General Medical Council (GMC) in 1996, the managers might consider referral to the GMC for a professional performance assessment. Also, with the introduction of clinical governance in the White Paper in 1997, new powers to compel further assessments may be introduced in the near future.

Case 3

The receptionist was in continuous employment with the employer for 3 years. Hence, she was not excluded from claiming unfair dismissal. If the 3-year fixed-term contract was such that it could not be terminated earlier except for a gross breach of contract by either the employer or the employee, then failure to renew the contract would constitute dismissal under the Employment Rights Act 1996.

The only question to answer is whether the dismissal was fair and reasonable. If the post was originally created because of extra work which was expected to last for 3 years, then it might be deemed reasonable. In this case, the employer went on to recruit another employee. Hence, it would be difficult for the employer to argue that it was reasonable. It appears likely that the receptionist could successfully claim unfair dismissal.

Case 4

As the ward sister had been in continuous employment for 3 years, she was qualified to claim unfair dismissal.

She left the post of her own accord without notice. However, as this was directly due to the employer's conduct which amounted to a breach of contract, she could claim that she was constructively dismissed. If the breach relates to an express term in the contract (e.g. change in the post or pay), then there would be little dispute that she would succeed. However, in this case, the ward sister would have to rely on an implied term (for the employer to treat employees with respect and trust). She might succeed if she was able to convince the tribunal of the facts, and that the conduct of the employer was so unreasonable as to amount to a breach of the contract.

Key points

• An employer can discipline an employee for a breach of the rules to which the employee's attention had been drawn previously.
• The rules may be general (this applies to all employer–employee relationships) or may be specific to the post.
• To be lawful:
  (a) the disciplinary procedures must be fair; and
  (b) the decisions must be reasonable.
• For minor offences, a step approach is recommended. Summary dismissal should be used only in extreme cases.
• Dismissal may be due to an employer's termination of contract, failure to renew a fixed-term contract or constructive dismissal.
• Constructive dismissal occurs when an employee leaves the post of his or her own volition as a result of the employer's unreasonable conduct amounting to significant breach of the contract.
• Disciplinary procedures for hospital doctors are governed by health circular HC(90)9, although new procedures are currently under consultation.
• In order to claim unfair dismissal, the employee must have a sufficient period of continuous employment, a dismissal must have taken place and it must have been unreasonable.

References

Brennan v. *Dewhurst Ltd* [1984] IRLR 629, EAT.
Department of Health (1999) *Supporting doctors, protecting patients. A consultation paper on preventing, recognising and dealing with poor clinical performance of doctors in England.* London: Department of Health.
Polkey v. *A. E. Dayton Services Ltd* [1988] AC 344.
Raymond B (1992) The Employment Rights of the NHS Hospital Doctor. In: Dyer C. (ed.) *Doctors, Patients and the Law.* Oxford: Blackwell Scientific Publications.
Robinson v. *Crompton Parkinson Ltd* [1978] IRLR 61.
Warner v. *Barbers Stores* [1978] IRLR 109.

Chapter 14 – Health and safety issues

In general, the law of health and safety at work mainly imposes responsibilities on employers:
- for all their employees; and
- for other people if their health and safety may be put at risk.

However, employees are also required:
- to take reasonable care for their own health and safety while at work; and
- to co-operate with employers in carrying out their duties.

Employers have always owed employees a duty of care under the common law (the law of negligence). The principles of the law of negligence are discussed in Chapter 9. However, since the Health and Safety at Work Act 1974 and subsequent legislation were passed, employers additionally owe employees a duty of care under these Acts of Parliament. The duty under these Acts resembles the common law duty in many ways, but is more stringent and detailed. Furthermore, whilst the law of negligence only gives rise to civil liability (i.e. it enables employees to claim compensation from their employers), the health and safety legislation mainly gives rise to criminal liability (i.e. it allows the Health and Safety Executive to issue improvement or prohibition notices or to prosecute those in breach of the legislation). However, since the conviction of a criminal offence may be used in civil proceedings (Civil Evidence Act 1968, section 11), the new legislation may also be relevant in civil proceedings. The focus of this chapter is on this new legislation.

The overall responsibility for administering the health and safety laws rests with the Health and Safety Commission. The enforcement of the Health and Safety at Work Act 1974 rests with the Health and Safety Executive. The environmental health officers of the local authorities also enforce the Act in some circumstances (e.g. in relation to food hygiene). The functions of the enforcement authorities include:
- appointing inspectors to inspect premises and collecting evidence for breaches of the legislation;
- serving improvement notices requiring employers to remedy the breaches;
- prohibiting certain activities in the premises for a certain period;
- seizing substances and items which may cause imminent danger; and
- prosecuting employers (either individuals or the organization).

The scope of the application of health and safety laws in the health services is extremely wide, and ranges from general issues (such as fire precaution and safety of doors and escalators) to very specific hazards (e.g. risks in handling particular drugs or infection risks). The specific health and safety issues may differ significantly amongst different health service settings. Furthermore, the issues in managing each specific risk tend to change very quickly with the introduction of new practices and technologies. Broadly speaking, three sets of rules are associated with the new legislation.

1 *The Act* contains a set of general rules which specify the persons made responsible.

2 *Regulations* are specific for each health and safety issue. These are made by the Secretary of State either on his or her own initiatives or on a proposal from the Health and Safety Commission.

3 *Codes of Practice* approved and issued by the Health and Safety Commission provide practical guidance on specific regulations. Other persons or organizations draw up a Code of Practice and submit it to the Commission for approval, and the codes may be continuously revised.

This chapter focuses on the general principles of the law relating to health and safety rather than the detailed regulations involved.

The general duties of employers to employees

Section 2 of the Health and Safety at Work Act 1974 places a duty on employers to ensure, as far as is reasonably practicable, the health, safety and welfare at work of all employees. In particular, it is the employer's duty to ensure safety and the absence of risks to the health of employees, as far as practicable, by:

1 providing and maintaining the place and systems of work;

2 making arrangements to ensure the safe use, handling, storage and transport of articles and substances;

3 ensuring the provision of information, instruction, training and supervision to both employees and, if necessary, to other non-employees;

4 maintaining any place of work and the means of access and egress which are under the employer's control; and

5 providing and maintaining facilities and arrangements for a safe working environment (e.g. freedom from noise and fumes, the provision of toilet facilities, etc.).

The following points should be noted.

1 Employers are expected to fulfil these duties only if it is reasonably practicable. What is reasonably practicable in a large organization (e.g. a hospital) may not be practicable in a smaller organization (e.g. a rural general practice).

2 Employers are only responsible for the safety of the premises over which they have actual control, but they may be responsible for a safe system of work on other premises. For example, GPs may have responsibility for safe policies when their practice nurses visit patients' homes, but may not have responsibility for risks due to deficiencies in the maintenance of the patients' homes.

3 In order to fulfil the duty in 3 above, all employers who employ five or more employees must:

    (a) prepare a written statement of their general policy on the health and safety at work of all employees and how the policy currently in force is carried out;

(b) revise the policy as frequently as is appropriate; and

(c) the policy should be brought to the attention of all their employees.

4 Regarding the duty to maintain a safe working environment, future regulations requiring most employers to enforce a no-smoking policy in the workplace are likely in view of recent strong evidence of harm from passive smoking.

Safety representatives and safety committee (section 2(4) (6) (7))

Safety representatives may be appointed from amongst employees who have 2 years of employment with the employer (or similar employment). The employer must consult with the safety representatives over a wide range of issues in order to facilitate employer–employee co-operation in developing measures to promote the health and safety at work of employees, and to check the effectiveness of these measures. The functions of the safety representatives include:

• investigating the potential hazards in the workplace and the causes of accidents;

• investigating complaints by employees relating to health and safety issues;

• making representations to employers on the above and other general matters;

• carrying out inspections;

• receiving information from health and safety inspectors of the Health and Safety Executive; and

• attending health and safety committee meetings. The employer must set up a safety committee if at least two safety representatives make such a request.

Employers must grant paid time off to employees who perform duties in relation to health and safety issues (e.g. safety representatives, members of safety committees, etc.) and these employees must not be disadvantaged as a result of participation in these activities (Employment Rights Act 1996, section 44, 100).

The general duties of employers to non-employees

Section 3 of the Health and Safety at Work Act 1974 imposes a duty on every employer to conduct his or her undertakings in such a way as to ensure, as far as is practicable, that persons not employed who may be potentially affected are not exposed to risks to their health or safety.

For example, in general practice, the principal GPs may be responsible for the health and safety of patients, students or other visitors to the practice. Similarly, a hospital trust may be responsible for the health and safety of patients, visitors, students and those working as independent contractors whilst on the premises. Any known potential hazard on the employer's premises must be communicated to these non-employees.

The general duties of employees

Sections 7 and 8 of the Health and Safety at Work Act 1974 impose a duty on employees while at work to:
• take reasonable care for the health and safety of themselves and others who may be affected by their acts or omissions at work;
• co-operate with employers to enable them to perform and comply with the duties imposed in relation to health and safety; and
• not to interfere with or misuse any equipment provided in the interests of health, safety or welfare (this also applies to non-employees).

   Successful prosecution of persons who are in breach of these duties may result in a fine. Employees may be subjected to disciplinary actions by their employers.

Key points

• The health and safety regulations exist to protect the health of employees (and non-employees).
• They mainly impose responsibility on employers to look after the health and safety of employees and non-employees.
• However, employees are also required to take reasonable care of their own health and safety, and to co-operate with their employers.
• Employers who breach the regulations may be prosecuted either as individuals or as an organization.
• The victim may also seek compensation through the civil courts.
• Employees who breach the regulations may also be prosecuted. They may also be subject to the employer's disciplinary actions.

Part 3
Legal Procedures

Death

After the death of a person, a doctor may be involved in one or more of the following processes:
1 confirming death;
2 arranging postmortem examinations;
3 arranging for tissues to be removed for transplantation;
4 issuing death certificates;
5 cremation procedures;
6 reporting the death to the coroner; and
7 writing a report for the coroner and/or attending the coroner's inquest.

Case 1

A 40-year-old man died after having been admitted to hospital 3 weeks previously with clinical features of congestive heart failure. A form of cardiomyopathy was strongly suspected clinically, although the precise type was not clear. The consultant in charge requested a postmortem examination. The senior house officer spoke to the deceased's wife who refused to permit the postmortem examination. The senior registrar in the clinical firm suggested that the senior house officer should inform the patient's wife that if she refused to allow the postmortem examination, the death would be reported to the coroner in order for a special postmortem to be carried out.

What would be the correct approach for the senior house officer? Could he or she issue a death certificate in the meantime?

Case 2

A 24-year-old man was admitted unconscious to the intensive care unit after a serious road traffic accident. He was ventilated, but his condition deteriorated 3 days later. He was unresponsive to deep pain. A neurologist and a neurosurgeon confirmed that he was brain-stem dead. The patient's mother informed the doctor that he had always wanted to donate his kidneys and cornea when he died. He intended to carry a donor card but had not done so. The patient's mother was also keen that his organs should be used for donation. The view of his father was not known, as he had not been in contact for over a year.

Whose consent was needed before the consultant could arrange for the organs to be removed for donation?

Case 3

Whilst on call on a Saturday night, Dr A, a pre-registration house physician, was called to confirm the death of a patient known to have cancer of the bronchus and who was under the care of another consultant, Dr B. Dr A had not seen the patient previously.

After the death was confirmed, the patient's relatives were very upset. Both the nursing staff and the relatives asked Dr A to write out the death certificate immediately so that they could arrange the funeral without further delay.

Could Dr A legally issue the death certificate?

As Dr A was unsure of the procedures, he declined to issue the death certificate, but documented his examination findings in the patient record. Dr C, Dr B's preregistration house officer, issued the death certificate on Monday morning. Three days later, Dr B was called to complete the relevant section on the cremation form.

Should Dr C have seen the body before issuing the death certificate? Should Dr B have seen the body before completing the medical certificate section of the cremation form?

Could Dr C complete the 'confirmatory medical certificate' section of the cremation form? Who may be eligible to complete this section? What should the person completing this section of the cremation form do?

Case 4

An 80-year-old woman had been diagnosed with carcinoma of the breast with metastasis for some time and died at home one evening. She was not seen by a doctor after her death. Her usual GP, Dr D, last saw the patient 3 weeks prior to her death. Dr D was asked to issue a death certificate.

Should Dr D inform the coroner? Could Dr D legally issue a death certificate? Could Dr D subsequently sign the medical certificate section of the cremation form?

Case 5

Should deaths due to the following causes be reported to the coroner? Is it likely that an inquest will be held? If so, what is the likely verdict at the inquest?

1 Meningococcal meningitis.
2 Acute alcohol withdrawal.
3 Death which occurred in the intensive care unit 12 hours after repair of an aortic aneurysm.
4 Acute hepatitis secondary to paracetamol overdose.
5 Pulmonary embolus secondary to deep vein thrombosis.
6 Following a serious road traffic accident.
7 Following a knife attack to the chest wall by a known mentally ill patient.

Comments on the case histories

Case 1

Under the Human Tissue Act 1961, the person in lawful possession of the body (i.e. the managers) must be satisfied that there are no objections to the postmortem examination from the relatives or the deceased prior to death. Hence, the consent of the patient's wife is essential before the examination is carried out.

The senior house officer could certainly issue the death certificate. The cause of death (i.e. congestive cardiac failure secondary to cardiomyopathy) was sufficiently specific for death certification purposes. Hence, the consultant's request for a postmortem examination was to investigate the precise nature and the extent of the disease.

Even if the doctors were entitled to report the death to the coroner, the coroner would be unlikely to perform a postmortem examination. Furthermore, it would be most inappropriate for the doctors to put pressure on the patient's relative into consenting to such an examination by threatening referral to the coroner.

The senior house officer should explain carefully to the patient's wife the nature of the postmortem examination, that such an examination might be beneficial to the family (e.g. if the type of cardiomyopathy was familial) and explore any fears which she might have. If she refused, the postmortem examination should not be pursued.

Case 2

Since a road traffic accident was the cause of death, the death must be reported to the coroner. Tissues must not be removed from the body without the coroner's consent. In practice, coroners seldom withhold consent. After the coroner's consent is given, the normal procedure should be followed.

Under the Human Tissue Act 1961, tissue may be removed after death for transplantation either:

1 if the deceased had given prior written consent or oral consent in the presence of two witnesses; or
2 if the person in lawful possession of the body (i.e. managers representing the health authority), after any reasonable enquiry as may be practicable, has no reason to believe that the deceased had ever expressed any objection to donation, or that the surviving relatives have made any such objection.

In this case, it is true that the deceased had not given valid prior consent. However, it would be sufficient to ascertain from his mother that the deceased had not expressed any objections to donation, and that no relatives have made any such objections before the manager or doctor representing the health authority authorizes the removal of tissue. The deceased's mother should be asked to sign the appropriate form.

Case 3

Dr A could not legally issue the death certificate, as he did not attend the patient during her last illness.

Although Dr C was not legally obliged to do so, it would be wise to view the body before signing the death certificate. Dr B was legally obliged to view the body before completing the medical certificate section of the cremation form.

Dr C should not complete the confirmatory medical certificate section of the cremation form, as Dr C worked in the same clinical department as Dr B who completed the medical certificate section. Another doctor who had been fully registered for more than 5 years and who was not in the same clinical department should complete the confirmatory medical certificate section. The doctor should view the body and question Dr B about the cause of death.

Case 4

Dr D must inform the coroner, as he had not attended the patient within 14 days prior to death.

Dr D could legally issue the death certificate. The 14 days rule, which applies to reporting death to the coroner, does not apply to issuing death certificates. However, he should initial Box A to indicate that the death had been reported to the coroner, and he should also view the body.

Dr D must not sign the medical certificate section of the cremation form until the coroner indicated that he intended to take no action by issuing Form A.

Case 5

The following deaths should be reported to the coroner.
2 Acute alcohol withdrawal.
3 Death which occurred in the intensive care unit 12 hours after repair of an aortic aneurysm.
4 Acute hepatitis secondary to paracetamol overdose.
6 Following a serious road traffic accident.
7 Following a knife attack to the chest wall by a known mentally ill patient.
Inquests are likely to be held for the following deaths.
6 Following a serious road traffic accident (probably without a jury).
7 Following a knife attack to the chest wall by a known mentally ill patient (probably with a jury, after the criminal procedures have been completed).
The verdict in 6 is likely to be 'accident', and the verdict in 7 is likely to be 'unlawful killing'.

Confirming death

For practical purposes, death is usually diagnosed by the absence of respiration and heartbeat. It is usually straightforward, and may be carried out by any fully registered doctor or by a pre-registration house officer. It is indicated by the absence of carotid pulses, the absence of heart sound on auscultation, the absence of respiratory movement and the breaking up of the blood columns in the retinal veins on examination of the optic fundi. Fixed non-reactive pupils may be a useful confirmatory sign. It is important that the doctor examines the patient carefully and for a sufficiently long time before pronouncing death. It is also important to write down the findings clearly in the patient's record. The heart rate may be slow, the pulse may be weak and the respiration may be shallow. Rarely, an electrocardiogram (ECG) or an electroencephalogram (EEG) may be useful. Death is sometimes wrongly diagnosed in barbiturate poisoning.

The diagnosis of death is considerably more difficult if the patient is artificially ventilated. For example, a patient may be artificially ventilated after a road traffic accident, but is subsequently thought to have suffered irreversible brain damage. Another example is the potential organ donor who is ventilated to maintain the viability of the donor organs.

There is no legal definition of death. However, the Conference of Royal College and Faculties of the United Kingdom issued a Code of Practice to diagnose brain death in 1979 and 1981. To summarize briefly, the patient must satisfy three initial criteria and must also satisfy several diagnostic brain-stem tests. The initial criteria are as follows.

1 The patient must be in deep coma which is not due to depressant drugs, hypothermia or metabolic disturbances.

2 The patient must be ventilated artificially due to inadequate or absent spontaneous respiration, and drugs (e.g. neuromuscular blocking agents) must be excluded as the cause.

3 The patient must have been clearly diagnosed with a disorder which can lead to brain death.

The diagnostic brain-stem tests must be repeated by two doctors who are independent of each other (the consultant in charge or a deputy with 5 or more years' experience, and another suitably experienced doctor). The tests must be carried out when the body temperature is higher than 35°C. The tests include pupillary responses, corneal reflexes, vestibulo-ocular reflexes, motor cranial responses, the gag reflex and spontaneous respiratory movement with a sufficiently high CO_2 level.

Brain-stem death is different from persistent vegetative state. Ethical dilemmas were highlighted in the case of Tony Bland (a victim at the Hillsborough football stadium in 1989) who was diagnosed as being in a persistent vegetative state. The House of Lords declared that it would not be unlawful to withdraw medical treatment (*Airedale NHS Trust* v. *Bland* 1993). In this condition, the brain-stem still functions, although all the cerebral cortical functions are lost. In the mid-1990s, mistakes in the diagnosis of persistent vegetative state were reported, and a consensus statement on the criteria for the persistent vegetative state is being developed (Jennett *et al.* 1997). However, it is important to note that patients in a persistent vegetative state are *not* legally dead.

Arranging postmortem examinations

If the cause of death is known and the death is not reportable to a coroner, a postmortem examination may still be desired for clinical or academic purposes to determine the extent of the disease process. In practice, it is also used to determine a more precise cause of death.

Under the Human Tissue Act 1961, the person who is lawfully in possession of the body may give permission for a postmortem examination if, having made as reasonable enquiry as may be practicable, he or she has no reason to believe that either the deceased person had indicated during life that he or she objected to such an examination, or any surviving relatives object to such an examination. The person lawfully in possession of the body in a hospital is usually the health authority responsible for the hospital. In practice, a form is given to the next-of-kin to sign to confirm the absence of objection to a postmortem examination, and a manager or doctor representing the health authority may then give permission for the examination. If death occurs outside the hospital, the person lawfully in possession of the body may be the next-of-kin or the executor of the will.

The law regarding the removal of limited amounts of tissue for research, teaching or therapeutic purposes is similar, and the next-of-kin may indicate the absence of objection on the same form.

Arranging for tissues to be removed for organ transplantation

Organ donors may be live donors or cadaver donors. For live donation, the risk to the life of the donor must be assessed. The procedure involved, the potential consequences and the risks must be explained fully to the donor. Written consent must be obtained in the presence of witnesses, and the donor must be encouraged to discuss the procedure with his or her family.

The Human Tissue Act 1961 also governs cadaver organ donation. Necessary permission for removal of tissues may be obtained in one of the following two ways.

1 *Prior consent given by the person before death (section 1).* This may be in writing or may have been given orally in the presence of two witnesses. In practice, carrying a signed donor card is the commonest way of indicating such consent.
2 *No consent given prior to death (section 2).* The procedures are very similar to those for postmortem examination. The person in lawful possession of the body (i.e. the health authority) may authorize the removal of donor tissue if, after as reasonable enquiry as may be practicable, he or she has no reason to believe that the deceased had ever expressed any objection to donation, or that the surviving relatives have made any such objection. In practice, discussion with one relative who has been in close contact with the deceased person previously would suffice. If the surviving relatives cannot be contacted, the health authority may still give permission.

For deaths reported to the coroner, additional permission from the coroner is required.

The removal of tissue must be performed by a fully, not provisionally, registered medical practitioner.

Future development: postmortem and organ retention

In 1999, there was a public outcry over disclosures that staff at Alder Hey Children's Hospital in Liverpool removed and stored, without the parents' explicit consent, more than 2000 hearts and 800 other organs from children who had undergone postmortem examination. Currently, organ retention is covered by the Human Tissue Act 1961, which allows the 'person lawfully in possession of the body' to authorize the removal of any part for research if he or she has no reason to believe that a relative objects.

As a result of scandals in Bristol where parents were shocked to find that organs from their children had been retained after postmortem examination without consultation, the Royal College of Pathologists published guidelines in March 2000 recommending that:

1 doctors seeking agreement for a postmortem examination must find out from the pathologists the necessity of and grounds for retaining tissues, so that relatives can make informed decisions;

2 for patients whose postmortem is required by coroners, the relatives should be given information leaflets on the legal necessity of postmortem, the need for tissue or organ retention (if appropriate), and their rights to the tissue or organ after the examination is completed. The postmortem report should state clearly what organs or tissues have been retained in pursuance of the investigation of the death; and

3 for patients whose postmortem is not requested by coroners, hospitals should make leaflets available for relatives containing detailed information on postmortem, organ or tissue retention, and their rights to grant or withhold consent. The consent form should give a range of options by which relatives can separately grant or withhold their agreements.

Issuing death certificates

The doctor who attended the patient during his or her last illness is legally obliged to issue the medical certificate of cause of death ('the death certificate'), irrespective of whether the death will be reported to the coroner (Births and Deaths Registration Act 1953). Hence, if the on-call junior doctor is asked to confirm the death of a patient who is looked after by another department, he or she should record the findings in the patient record, but the doctor who usually looks after the patient should issue the death certificate the following working day. Similarly, if a GP confirms the death of a patient who is looked after by another practice whilst on call in the evening, the GP who looked after the patient most recently should issue the death certificate.

Even if the death is to be reported to the coroner, it is still necessary to consider whether to issue a death certificate. On a practical level, it would be difficult for the doctor to issue a death certificate if he or she could not specify a probable cause of death. The death should be reported to the coroner. However, if the doctor is able to specify a probable cause of death, though not to a high degree of certainty, a death certificate should be issued and the death should be reported to the coroner. Box A of the death certificate should be initialled to indicate that the death has been reported to the coroner. The doctor can issue a death certificate even though a postmortem has been requested. Box B should be initialled to indicate that additional information as to the cause of death may be available later. Although not legally obliged to do so, it may be wise for the doctor to view the body.

The death certificate details the name of the deceased, the date of death, place of death, time last seen, the causes of death and whether the death might have been contributed to by the employment of the deceased. The causes of death are divided into Part I (disease or condition directly leading to death) and Part II (other significant conditions contributing to the death but not relating to the condition causing it). Part I itself may be divided into I(a), I(b) and I(c)—I(a) is due to I(b), which in turn is due to I(c). An example is: I(a) renal failure, I(b) ureteric obstruction and I(c) carcinoma of the cervix; Part II hypertension.

Certificate of disposal

The death certificate is given to the 'informant'. For deaths which occur in houses and public institutions, the informant may be a relative of the deceased who was present at the death, attended the last illness or resided with the deceased, the occupier of the house, or the hospital administrator. For deaths which do not occur in houses or public institutions, any relative of the deceased, any person present at the death or any person who found or is in charge of the body may be the informant.

The informant must take the death certificate to the Registrar's Office, in addition to other documents such as the medical card and the pension book. If there are no irregularities in the documents, the Registrar will issue and deliver a certificate for disposal to the undertaker. If the body is to be cremated, the cremation procedures should be followed. The funeral director will inform the Registrar once disposal is complete.

Cremation

In the UK, almost three-quarters of dead bodies are cremated. The cremation procedures are based on the Cremation Act 1902. To apply for cremation, no less than four persons need to complete the prescribed forms as follows.

1 Form A—(application: to be completed by a relative or the executor of the will, and countersigned by a person of good repute). To confirm that the deceased had no objection to cremation and that there is no reason to believe that death was due to any unnatural cause.

2 Form B—(medical certificate: to be completed by the doctor who issued the death certificate). The doctor *must* have viewed the body after death. (If the death certificate is issued by the coroner, Form E will be completed by the coroner instead.)

3 Form C—(confirmatory medical certificate: to be completed by a doctor who has been fully registered for at least 5 years, and who is not working as a partner in a practice or in the same clinical department as the doctor completing Form B). The doctor should view the body after death and question the doctor who completed Form B. (Again, if the death certificate is issued by the coroner, Form E completed by the coroner would suffice.)

4 Form F—(authority to cremate: to be completed by the medical referee, usually a community or public health medicine doctor).

Reporting the death to the coroner

Who are coroners?

The role of the coroner has diminished in the last 900 years, and the coroner is now mainly responsible for investigating deaths. There are about 150 coroners in England and Wales. Coroners are solicitors, barristers or doctors of at least 5 years' experience in their professions, although most are considerably more experienced. In recent years, most coroners have been lawyers. In the London districts, many coroners are both medically and legally qualified. Coroners are employed by the local authorities and they have much autonomy in discharging their duty.

Who reports deaths to the coroner?

Strictly speaking, only the Registrar of Births and Deaths has a legal duty to report deaths to the coroner. In practice, most cases are reported by doctors and the police.

Which deaths should be reported to the coroner?

The Registrar automatically refers the following death certificates to the coroner, and doctors should refer these deaths to the coroner before the death certificates are issued:

• death of a person who was not attended by a doctor in his or her last illness;
• death of a person who was not seen by a doctor either within 14 days before death or after death;

- when the cause of death is not known;
- deaths due to industrial disease;
- deaths due to poisoning;
- suspicious or probable unnatural deaths;
- deaths due to violence, neglect or abortion; and
- deaths which occur during a surgical operation or before recovery from an anaesthetic.

In addition, the following deaths should also be reported:
- deaths which occur within 24 hours of emergency admission;
- deaths associated with medical treatment (e.g. deaths which occur within 24 hours of a surgical operation);
- deaths for which medical negligence is alleged;
- deaths which occur in prisons and police custody;
- homicides, suicides and accidents;
- infant deaths (including stillbirths);
- deaths due to hypothermia;
- deaths due to chronic alcoholism; and
- deaths associated with drug dependence.

What are the procedures for reporting deaths to the coroner?

Deaths should be reported by telephone to the coroner officer, who is usually an experienced police officer. The police officer will gather details of the deceased and the circumstances leading to the death, and the papers prepared will be studied by the coroner. The coroner may take one of the two following options.

1 *No postmortem examination required.* If the coroner is satisfied that the doctor who attended the last illness of the deceased knows the cause of death and a postmortem examination is not required, he may inform the Registrar of Births and Deaths by issuing Form A. The doctor who attended the deceased's last illness may then issue the death certificate.

2 *Postmortem examination required.* If the coroner is not satisfied that the cause of death is known, he will request a pathologist to perform a postmortem examination. If this reveals natural causes of death, he will inform the Registrar of Births and Deaths of the cause of death by issuing Form B, and the body may be disposed. If the postmortem examin-ation reveals probable unnatural causes of death, an inquest will be held to determine the cause of death.

Deaths for which an inquest is usually held include:
- deaths which are possibly due to homicide. If it appears that a criminal prosecution is likely, the coroner will forward the papers to the Crown Prosecution Service and adjourn the inquest hearing until after the criminal trial;
- deaths due to suicide;
- deaths caused by traffic accidents;

- deaths caused by industrial accidents or disease;
- deaths in prison or police custody;
- deaths due to neglect; and
- deaths where medical negligence has been alleged.

The inquest

The only purpose of an inquest is to determine the identity of the deceased, as well as where, when and how the death occurred. It is not concerned with determining criminal or civil liability, or with apportioning blame.

The coroner may hold an inquest with or without a jury. The coroner must sit with a jury for deaths caused by industrial accidents, deaths caused by accidents in ships, rail or aircraft and deaths in prison or police custody, although the coroner may choose to sit with a jury in other cases.

The doctors who attended the deceased are asked to prepare medical reports for the coroner before the inquest. If the reports are not disputed by the relatives or other interested parties, they are usually accepted as documentary evidence and the doctors are not called to give evidence orally. Otherwise, the doctors will be summoned to give evidence at the inquest.

The relatives may be represented by solicitors or barristers, although this is rare unless medical or industrial negligence is alleged. Doctors may also be represented by medical defence organizations, solicitors or barristers. They should always inform their medical defence organization if the question of medical negligence may be raised at all, as evidence given at the inquest may be used in subsequent negligence claims in the civil court. During the inquest, documentary evidence is produced and witnesses are examined. The coroner ensures that only admissible evidence is taken into account. The examination of witnesses is similar to other legal proceedings. However, the inquest differs from other legal proceedings in many ways. As the inquest is a fact-finding rather than an adversarial exercise, there are no opening or closing speeches by the parties, and the procedures are slightly less strict and formal.

The possible verdicts of an inquest include:
- natural causes;
- unlawful killing;
- suicide;
- accidental death or misadventure;
- dependence upon a drug;
- neglect; and
- open verdict (i.e. there was insufficient information to determine the nature of the death—the inquest may be resumed at a later date if more information comes to light.

Key points

Diagnosing death

• Deaths associated with the absence of respiration and heartbeat can be diagnosed by any one doctor.
• The diagnosis of brain-stem death requires two independent, experienced doctors following a more complicated set of procedures.
• Persistent vegetative state is not legally death.

Postmortem examination not requested by a coroner

• The purpose is to determine the extent of the disease process.
• This may be authorized if, after reasonable enquiries, there is no reason to believe that either the deceased had ever expressed objection or the surviving relatives have any objections.
• The death certificate may be issued after the postmortem examination is completed by initialling Box B.

Arranging for tissues to be removed for transplantation

• This may be authorized if either:
  (a) the deceased had given valid consent before death; or
  (b) there is no reason to believe that the deceased had ever expressed objections or that the surviving relatives object.
• Deaths reported to the coroner require additional consent from the coroner.

Issuing death certificates

• Death certificates are usually issued by the doctor who attended the deceased's last illness.
• If a probable cause of death is known, the death certificate can be issued even if the death is reported to the coroner or a postmortem examination has been requested.
• The death certificate is usually given to a relative, who takes it to the Registrar's Office. A certificate of disposal is issued if the documents are in order.

Cremation

• In the UK, almost three-quarters of all dead bodies are cremated.

- Form B (the medical certificate section) is completed by the doctor who issued the death certificate.
- Form C (the confirmatory medical certificate section) is completed by an experienced doctor independent of the doctor who signs Form B.
- Both doctors must have viewed the body after death.

Reporting deaths to the coroner

- If the deceased was not seen by a doctor within 14 days prior to death, the death should be reported to the coroner.
- The coroner may or may not require a postmortem examination.
- If the coroner requests a postmortem examination, an inquest may or may not be held.

The inquest

- The inquest is a fact-finding procedure to determine the identity of the deceased, and when, where and how the death occurred.
- The procedures for examination of witnesses are similar to other legal proceedings.
- Relatives and doctors may or may not be legally represented.
- If an allegation of medical negligence is a possibility, the doctor should inform the medical defence organization before submitting a report to the coroner.

References

Airedale NHS Trust v. *Bland* [1993] AC 789.

Jennett B, Cranford R, Zasler N (1997) Consensus statement on criteria for the persistent vegetative state is being developed. *British Medical Journal* 314, 1621.

Knight B (1997) *Legal Aspects of Medical Practice*, 5th edition. Edinburgh: Churchill Livingstone.

Royal College of Pathologists (March 2000) Guidelines for the retention of tissues and organs at postmortem examinations.

Chapter 16 – Research and publications

Health professionals who engage in research usually have to take the following steps:
1 writing a research proposal: this includes stating the research question, the research design and protocol;
2 considering how to recruit and obtain consent from research subjects;
3 obtaining approval from relevant bodies (e.g. local research ethics committee);
4 carrying out the research; and
5 publishing and disseminating the research results.
In going through the various stages, they may encounter the following practical legal and ethical issues:
• general principles of obtaining valid consent from the research participants;
• obtaining approval from research ethics committees and relevant licensing requirements; and
• obtaining data and publishing research results without breaching confidentiality.

General principles of obtaining valid consent from the research participants

The appropriate consent to be obtained depends on several factors:
• the level of participation involved;
• whether the participant has capacity to consent;
• whether the participant is a patient or a volunteer; and
• if the participant is a patient, whether patients are expected to derive direct benefits from the research (i.e. therapeutic or non-therapeutic benefits).

The level of participation involved

The level of consent required increases with the level of participation. In general, if research involves physical contact with patients, explicit consent is required, as otherwise it would constitute battery.

Research which does not include active involvement, physical contact with patients or divulging identifiable data from patients to a third party might not require explicit consent if certain conditions are met. An example is a research project to find the prevalence of a disease within the population from computer records. The local research ethics committee should assess the conditions under which the research is to be carried out, and the following are generally regarded as the minimum:
• access to the clinical record is essential for the research and consent is not practicable;

- the research has sufficient scientific merit;
- the research may benefit the category of patients whose records are studied;
- it is not anticipated that contact will be made with the patients as a result of research findings;
- access is restricted to specific categories of information necessary for the research;
- permission is obtained from the clinicians and administrators responsible for the patients' care; and
- the rules on confidentiality should be followed.

Research that requires the active involvement of the patient requires fully informed consent. The general concept of informed consent is explained in Chapter 1. The broad nature of the procedures and the possible side-effects of the intervention must be explained to the patients fully. It would appear that the duty to explain is more important for research participants than for patients given recognized medical treatments, although there is no explicit legal authority on this point.

It is public policy that research participants must not be placed at unacceptable risk, even with their fully informed consent. One of the roles of the research ethics committees and the drug licensing regulations is to ensure that participants are not exposed to unacceptable risk.

Whether the participant has capacity to consent

Children and incompetent adults may pose difficulties in obtaining valid consent. It is practically difficult to obtain consent from them, and some would argue that they should not be subjects of research. On the other hand, some conditions are specific to children and those with mental disorders, for example, and it would otherwise be difficult to advance knowledge of these conditions. It is necessary to balance the need to obtain fully informed consent with the good of the public in order to carry out the research.

Children

For medical treatment, children above 16 years of age or children under 16 years who are sufficiently mature to understand the nature of the treatment may give legally valid consent themselves. For children under 16 years who are not sufficiently mature, those with parental responsibility can give legally valid consent.

For research purposes, these general rules hold good for children above 16 years. It would also appear that children under 16 years who are sufficiently mature to understand the nature of the research may give legally valid consent themselves, although there are no legal authorities on this point. However, they need to understand what research is, the purpose of the research and whether they are likely to benefit directly from it. Children may need to have more mature understanding to consent to research compared to children receiving medical treatment.

For children below 16 years who are not sufficiently mature to understand the nature of the research, the issue is more complicated. Whether those with parental responsibility can give legally valid consent depends on many factors. Generally speaking, they can only give legally valid consent if it is in the best interests of the child, and reasonable parents would consent under similar situations. The following factors are important:

• whether there are any direct benefits to the child—the greater the likely direct benefits, the more likely that the parents may give legally valid consent; and
• the degree of risks involved—the lower the risks, the more likely that they will give legally valid consent.

Even if parents may give legally valid consent, it would be good clinical practice for the researchers to inform the child as fully as practicable of what is involved in the research.

Mentally incapacitated adults

Currently in England and Wales, no one may give legally valid consent for medical treatment to mentally incapacitated adults. Even the courts cannot give such consent, although they have, on application from clinicians, declared that specific medical treatments given without consent were not illegal.

Obtaining legally valid consent for research is even more difficult. For therapeutic research (i.e. where the patient may derive direct benefits), it may be argued that participating in research is in the best interests of the patient. For non-therapeutic research, there are strong arguments for not carrying it out at all. The Medical Research Council (MRC) argued from a public policy point of view that non-therapeutic research can sometimes be justified if it may benefit a particular category of incapacitated people, and that the risks are minimal. However, this has not been tested in the courts.

Difficult issues in obtaining consent for research

Randomized controlled trials

In order to obtain scientifically valid results, the research protocol must be designed to avoid bias. In evaluating which of the two treatments is more effective, one potential source of bias is that clinicians may be more likely to allocate patients with more serious illness to one type of treatment than the other type. The randomized controlled trial (RCT) is designed to avoid this bias. In an RCT, the actual treatment the patient receives is determined by a randomizing scheme. Ideally, the clinicians and the patients themselves should not know which type of treatment is being given (i.e. it is a double-blind trial). In this way, sources of bias are minimized.

Whilst this type of research protocol would yield the most scientifically valid results, it poses a dilemma in obtaining informed consent. The clinician cannot choose the type of treatment which he or she considers to be best for the patient, and the clinician may not even know about the treatment the patient is receiving. It would not be difficult to inform the patient of the type of treatment he or she is receiving. Hence, it would not be possible to explain all the side-effects fully and frankly.

The argument in favour of performing an RCT is that the benefits to the general public may outweigh the difficulty of obtaining fully informed consent. It is also argued that the necessity for carrying out an RCT means that the balance of opinion about the alternative treatments is in equipoise. That is, as it is not known which of the treatments is better, prescribing one or the other treatment can both be said to be in the patient's best interests.

However, this type of argument may not hold for several reasons. Firstly, the patient may have known characteristics (e.g. previous medical illnesses) which favour the use of one type of treatment over another. Secondly, alternative treatments in RCTs are not always truly in equipoise. Existing evidence may favour one treatment over another in observational studies, but RCTs are required to confirm this. Thirdly, even if the treatments are equally effective, patients may prefer one type of treatment to another because of social and personal preferences. They are denied this choice in an RCT. Fourthly, it would not be easy to obtain fully informed consent practically, as many patients would find it hard to grasp the concept of randomization.

Obtaining approval from research ethics committees and relevant licensing requirements

Research in the NHS: the local research ethics committees

To decide whether a given research proposal is ethical, it would be necessary to assess its scientific merits, the design and performance of the research, as well as the procedures for obtaining appropriate consent from the subjects. It would be difficult for researchers to assess their own research proposals and progress objectively. In order to ensure that medical research is carried out both ethically and legally, research ethics committees have been established since 1968 to approve research proposals and to oversee medical research carried out on NHS patients. Most health authorities have now established their own local research ethics committees.

The Department of Health (1991) recommends that local research ethics committees should have between 8 and 12 members. They should include hospital medical staff, nursing staff, GPs and two or more lay people. Both sexes and a wide range of age groups should be represented. The members should be drawn to provide a sufficiently broad range of experience and expertise, so that the scientific and medical aspects of research proposals can be considered, taking the welfare of research subjects into consideration.

According to the Department of Health guidelines in 1991, approval must be sought from the local research ethics committee if the research involves:
• NHS patients (including those treated under contracts with private sector providers);
• fetal material and *in vitro* fertilization involving NHS patients;
• patients who have recently died on NHS premises;
• the access to records of past or present NHS patients; and
• the use of NHS premises or facilities.

However, the local research ethics committee may also advise on research outside the NHS (e.g. research carried out by universities or the MRC).

Research ethics committees should consider at least the following factors in a research proposal:
• the assessment of the scientific merits of the proposal;
• the effect on the health of the research subjects;
• any possible hazards to the research subjects and whether there are sufficient facilities available to deal with them;
• the degree of discomfort or mental distress foreseen;
• the adequacy of the research, and the qualifications and experience of the supervisor;
• any conflicts of interests involved, e.g. financial or other inducements offered to interested parties;
• the procedures for obtaining consent from research subjects or parents;
• whether appropriate information sheets for subjects have been prepared;
• procedures for monitoring research as it progresses;
• whether there are arrangements for ex-gratia compensation in case of injuries to research subjects.

Multicentre research ethics committees (MREC)

To ensure sufficient subjects are recruited, research has been increasingly carried out simultaneously in several centres. This has resulted in several problems. Firstly, researchers experience considerable delay in obtaining approval from all the relevant local research ethics committees. Secondly, different local research ethics committees may make different amendments to the research protocol which may prove to be incompatible.

The Department of Health carried out a review of multicentre research in 1997. An MREC will be established in every English region, and one each in

Wales, Scotland and Northern Ireland. Any research carried out within five or more local research ethics committee's geographical boundaries will be considered 'multicentred'. Such multicentre research protocols will be considered by one MREC only, usually in the region where the principal researcher is based. The MREC will give advice to the local research ethics committees involved. Once the MREC approves a research protocol, each local research ethics committee will be able either to accept or reject the proposal for local reasons. However, they are not allowed to amend the protocol.

Research with special licensing requirements

Pharmaceutical research (regulated by the Medicines Control Agency)
The Medicines Control Agency (part of the Department of Health) is responsible for licensing drugs. Drugs are required to undergo a lengthy testing process before they are licensed for use in humans. Firstly, the research is carried out in animals. If the results are favourable, the drugs may be tested in humans as follows.

• *Phase 1 trial*: the dosages at which the drugs can be tolerated are tested in healthy volunteers. They need to be approved by the local research ethics committee.
• *Phase 2 trial*: to test for clinical effects of drugs at doses shown to be tolerable in the phase 1 trial. A clinical trial certificate or appropriate exemptions from the Medicines Control Agency are required.
• *Phase 3 trial*: to compare the clinical benefits identified in phase 2 with existing treatments. A clinical trial certificate or appropriate exemptions from the Medicines Control Agency are required.
• *Product licence*: if the drug is shown to be effective, the drug company may apply to the Medicines Control Agency for a product licence. Drugs may continue to be tested in trials after licensing (phase 4 trial).

Human embryology research (regulated by the Human Fertilization and Embryology Authority)
Licences must be obtained from the Human Fertilization and Embryology Authority for research on human embryos. The project and the premises on which the project is carried out must be licensed. The Authority has strict guidelines on the issue of licences and a licence would not be granted unless it is absolutely necessary to use embryos for the research.

Research involving the administration of a radioactive medicinal product
A special certificate is required under the Medicines (Administration or Radioactive Substances) Regulations 1978.

Obtaining data and publishing research results without breaching confidentiality

Obtaining data without breaching confidentiality

Unless the patient has explicitly stated otherwise, consent for the research does not authorize patient-identifiable data to be made known to a third party other than the clinician. Hence, data should be made anonymous (patient non-identifiable) before they are given to researchers and their assistants.

Making the data anonymous requires careful consideration, as removing the patients' names alone does not always make them non-identifiable. For example, the patient can be easily identified if his or her postal address, age and sex are included in the data.

All those who have access to the data should be instructed in the importance of keeping the patient's information confidential. The clinician may need to be ultimately responsible for any breaches of confidentiality.

Publishing research results without breaching confidentiality

A few years ago, patients' clinical photographs and laboratory results were often published in books and journals without their consent. There have been complaints from patients recently when data (e.g. clinical photographs, X-ray film and laboratory results) which may identify the individuals were published.

The General Medical Council (GMC) has recently proposed guidelines stating that clinicians should obtain consent from patients before publishing personal information about them as individuals in journals, textbooks or other media in the public domain, whether or not the clinicians believe that the patients could be identified. Most major journals are now following these guidelines and will refuse to publish patients' information without their written consent.

The *British Medical Journal* has given the following situations when the rule may be relaxed.
• The patient is long dead and has no living relatives.
• The interaction with the patient was long ago (e.g. more than 15 years).
• The interaction was long ago and the patient was elderly or terminally ill, so the patient is likely to be dead.
• The material is to be published without the authors' names attached, so that it is unlikely anyone would be able to identify the patient.
• Even if the patient were to identify him- or herself, the events described are unlikely to cause offence.
• In sections of the journal where authors may fictionalize material.
It must be noted that these occasions arise rarely. In obtaining consent from patients for publications, the nature and purpose of the publication must be

clearly explained to them. Ideally, the proposed manuscript should be shown to the patient.

Case 1

Nurse A worked as a research associate in a university and was engaged to carry out research into any possible causal relationship between stomach cancer and alcohol consumption. She proposed to conduct a retrospective case–control study by extracting and analysing data from the medical records of over 2000 patients in a teaching hospital who were known to have developed the cancer, and controls who did not develop the cancer. It would not be necessary to interview, examine, investigate or alter the management of any patients.

What steps should she take to obtain consent? What practical steps should she take before performing the research?

Case 2

A surgeon at a teaching hospital would like to conduct an RCT to determine whether it is more clinically effective to perform cholecystectomy by an open operation or by the laparoscopic method on a certain subgroup of patients. Patients in a given subgroup of patients who required cholecystectomy would be randomized to have their gallbladders removed either by open surgery or by the laparoscopic method. Whilst there are some published studies comparing the two methods in the general population, it is not clear which of the methods would be more effective in the subgroup of patients being studied.

What information should the surgeon give to the patients before recruiting them to the study? What practical steps should he take before performing the research?

Case 3

A 2-year-old boy was suffering from a rare form of neuroblastoma (cancer of the adrenal medulla) and was admitted to a teaching hospital under the care of a paediatric oncologist and surgeon. A new regimen of chemotherapy had been tried in several other patients in the unit and appeared to be effective, and the oncologist wanted to perform a formal trial comparing its effectiveness with the usual chemotherapy regimen used in the hospital.

How should the oncologist obtain valid consent for the patient to enter the trial?

Case 4

Dr B was carrying out research into the antibody responses to a new chickenpox vaccine. He proposed immunizing half the children in a certain school who had no chickenpox antibody and re-measuring their antibody responses after a few weeks. He easily obtained parental consent for this. However, he also wished to re-measure the antibody levels of children who had not received the vaccine a few weeks later to ensure that there had not been a recent subclinical chickenpox epidemic.

Can the parents of children who had not received the vaccine give valid consent to this?

Case 5

Dr C, a psychiatrist and psychologist, developed certain 'cognitive training courses', and proposed researching into their possible benefits for patients with moderately severe dementia.

How may Dr C obtain valid consent for this research?

Case 6

A 45-year-old man was a victim of an armed robbery and suffered gunshot wounds to his head. The details of the armed robbery were reported on national television and news programmes. He was admitted to hospital where neurosurgeons successfully employed an innovative neurosurgical technique to treat his injury, but unfortunately he died of pulmonary embolus a few days later. The neurosurgeons wished to publish a case report with full clinical details including radiological films in a leading national medical journal. They argued that this should be permissible as long as the patient's name was not published.

Is this true?

Analysis of case histories

Case 1

The research proposed by nurse A required access to patients' records, but would not require any active involvement of the patients. Strictly speaking, patients' consent is essential for any type of research. However, obtaining explicit consent from all 2000 patients would be practically very difficult. Hence, it can be argued that explicit consent from patients may be dispensed with if the research project is scientifically sound and may benefit future patients with stomach cancer. The local research ethics committee would assess the scientific merits of the research proposal. Nurse A should demonstrate the scientific merits in her research proposal to the local research ethics committee. It is essential that nurse A obtains permission from the clinicians in charge and the medical records department for access to the patients' records. Nurse A and all her assistants must keep all patients' information confidential.

Case 2

The surgeon should inform the patients that their condition requires a chole-cystectomy, and should explain all the risks involved in both methods of chole-cystectomy. He should inform the patients what he believes to be the relative effectiveness of the two treatments from current evidence. He should then explain the concept of randomization, the fact that the patients will be allocated to one of the two treatments and the reasons behind it. The patients should be asked to sign a consent form if they agree to participate in the trial.

Case 3

Clearly, a 2-year-old boy would not be able to understand the nature of the proposed treatment and consent should be obtained from those with parental responsibility. The main issue is whether his parents can give legally valid consent for the research, assuming that the local research ethics committee has approved the research project. The research proposed is therapeutic (i.e. the patient can be expected to directly benefit from it). Although there may be risks involved, it can be said that reasonable parents could be expected to consent under similar circumstances. Hence, the consent from those with parental responsibility would be legally valid.

Case 4

The children who did not receive the vaccination would be unlikely to benefit directly from the re-measurement of their antibody levels, as their antibody levels would be unlikely to change over a few weeks. However, it can be argued that the risks involved in re-measurement are minimal, and it can be said that reasonable parents could be expected to consent under similar circumstances. Hence, the consent from those with parental responsibility would be legally valid.

Case 5

It would be impossible for Dr C to obtain legally valid consent. The patient clearly would not be mentally competent to give informed consent. Currently, relatives cannot give legally valid consent on behalf of mentally incompetent adults. It is most unlikely that the patient would have given a valid advance directive.

The research can be carried out only if it can be argued that participation is in the patient's best interests. A case may be made out if there is substantial evidence that the treatment may benefit the patient. The local research ethics committee would assess the evidence before approving the research proposal.

Case 6

The main issue is whether publication would lead to a breach of confidentiality. The fact that the patient has died does not affect the clinician's duty to confidentiality.

It is not true that the clinician can publish the clinical details of the patient as long as his name is omitted. The main issue is whether the material is patient-identifiable, i.e. whether readers (e.g. the patient's friends) could identify the patient by reading the case history. Given the wide coverage of the armed robbery incident in the press, it is likely that the readers would be able to identify the patient unless the clinical details were carefully worded. In any case, most major journals would not publish the case history unless they were certain that the patient could not be identified from the article.

Although not a legal requirement, it would be good clinical practice to obtain consent for the proposed publication from the relatives of the deceased patient.

Key points

General principles of obtaining valid consent from research participants

• Fully informed consent must be obtained from research participants.
• The level of consent is higher for non-therapeutic research (i.e. if participants cannot be expected to derive direct benefits) than for therapeutic research.
• If active participation is not required, explicit consent might be dispensed with if the research has scientific and medical merit, and consent cannot be obtained practically.

Children

• Generally, those with parental responsibility may give legally valid consent if reasonable parents could be expected to consent under similar conditions.
• Parents may generally give consent for therapeutic research.
• Parents may give consent for non-therapeutic research only if the potential risks to the child are minimal.

Mentally incapacitated adults

• Currently, no one can give legally valid consent on behalf of mentally incapacitated adults.
• Therapeutic research is justified only if it is in the best interests of the subject (i.e. the subject is likely to benefit directly from it).
• Very strong arguments are needed to carry out non-therapeutic research.

Practical considerations

Obtaining approval from research ethics committees

• All research carried out on NHS patients or on patients treated in NHS premises requires approval from the research ethics committee.

• Before approving a research proposal, the research ethics committee considers issues such as the scientific merits, the design of the protocol, supervision and participants' consent.
• For research involving five or more local research ethics committee's geographical boundaries, the protocol should first be approved by the multicentre research ethics committee.

Licensing requirements

There are special licensing requirements for research:
• on development;
• on new drugs;
• on embryos; and
• involving administration of radioactive medicinal substances.

Insurance against negligence claims

• Where appropriate, those engaged in research should check with the medical defence organizations whether the proposed research is covered.

Confidentiality

• All researchers and their assistants should keep all participants' information confidential.
• The clinician in charge of a project should ensure that all researchers and their assistants are aware of this duty.
• If possible, researchers should be given non-patient-identifiable data.
• Publication of potentially patient-identifiable clinical details (including photographs or radiographs) in books or journals usually requires explicit consent from patients. Whether the information is patient-identifiable should be carefully assessed.

References

Doyal L (1997) Informed consent in medical research: Journals should not publish research to which patients have not given fully informed consent—with three exceptions. *British Medical Journal* 314: 1107–11.
Kelly G (1998) Patient data, confidentiality, and electronics. *British Medical Journal* 316: 718–19.
Smith R (1998) Informed consent: edging forwards (and backwards). *British Medical Journal* 316: 949–51.

Chapter 17 – Writing medico-legal reports and giving evidence in court

Writing medico-legal reports

Introduction

Many health professionals will be asked to write medico-legal reports and doctors are frequently asked to do so. Occasionally, the writing of the report may be followed by a court appearance when the doctor is asked to give evidence. Doctors are asked to write medico-legal reports by different agents, e.g. insurance companies, solicitors, the police, etc. These reports may serve different purposes, e.g. for administrative purposes, for criminal prosecution, for personal injury claims, for medical negligence claims or to determine the cause of death. How the report should be written depends on its purpose.

Doctors may be asked to write a purely factual report as a professional witness. Here, the doctor has seen the patient professionally, and is asked to give a description of the patient's symptoms and signs, the diagnosis and the treatment. On the other hand, doctors may also be asked to give an opinion as an expert witness. In this case, the doctor may or may not have previously seen the patient, and he or she is asked to provide expert medical opinion.

When a doctor is asked to write a report, two questions should be clarified.

1 Who requests the report and what is the purpose?
2 Has the patient given consent, or is consent required?

The person requesting the report and the purpose of the report

Examples of people requesting reports and their purposes are:
• solicitors representing the patient, e.g. in personal injury or medical negligence claims;
• solicitors representing health authorities or Trusts, e.g. in defending medical negligence claims;
• insurance companies, e.g. to decide on the terms of an insurance policy;
• employers, e.g. to confirm that the employee is fit to take up employment;
• tribunals, e.g. to determine the entitlement of patients to benefits; and
• coroners, to determine the cause of death.

The form and content of the report depend heavily on its purpose. It is important to answer the questions raised by the enquirer and to exclude irrelevancies. Hence, it is important to clarify at the outset the questions the enquirer wants answered and whether one is asked to act as a professional witness or an expert witness.

The patient's consent

Before writing the report, it is important to ensure that the patient has given consent to the disclosure of the medical information and, if the report is for insurance or employment purposes, the procedures in the Access to Medical Reports Act 1988 are fulfilled (see Chapter 4). Usually, the person requesting the report obtains consent from the patient, but the health professional should check that this consent has been obtained, and that the patient knows the purpose of the report. A coroner's request for a report on a death within his or her jurisdiction must be complied with. However, a request from the police for a report need not be complied with unless the patient's consent is obtained, or in extreme cases, where the public interest overrides private interest for confidentiality.

After the report has been written, one should ensure that no one else other than the person requesting the report has access to it. If the report is requested in contemplation of litigation, it is important that a copy is not kept in the medical records. Such reports may be exempt from disclosure to other parties, but the production of the medical records may be applied for by other parties.

The form and content of the report

All reports should be word-processed, with a clear layout. The precise form and content of the report depend on several factors:
- whether one acts as a professional or expert witness;
- the specialty involved; and
- the purpose for which the report is prepared.

The report is targeted at an educated person with no previous medical training. Hence, the meaning of any medical or scientific terms must be made clear. The language used should be precise and medical jargon should be avoided as far as possible. It is important that health professionals write the report impartially and avoid undue influence by the patient or the lawyers instructing them. Health professionals have a duty to the court and must provide a report which reflects the full picture of the case. It must be remembered that there is always a possibility that the health professional will be asked to appear in court at a later date to be asked about the contents of the report and that he or she might regret a carelessly written report.

Report from a professional witness

It must be stressed from the outset that if there is any hint of criticism of the health professional's management in the case, advice should be sought from his or her defence organizations or unions before sending out any reports.

A professional witness usually reports on the previous consultation by and treatment of a patient with whom he or she had direct clinical involvement. Hence, a large part of the report would be factual, detailing the history, examination findings, investigational results and the treatments given. There may be a small part of the report giving an opinion on the cause of the condition and the prognosis of the patient.

A professional witness report should include the following information.

1 *Introduction.*
   (a) The date when the report was written.
   (b) The purpose for which the report was written.
   (c) The date, place and the circumstances of the patient's consultation.
   (d) The source of the patient's referral.

2 *Clinical history, examination and management.*
All relevant information should be included and presented logically. This usually begins with the clinical history and examination findings, the investigative results, and the treatments given. The source of the information should be made clear in the clinical history, especially if criminal or civil litigation is involved. For example, say 'the patient said the injuries were sustained when he was attacked by two youths ...' rather than 'the patient suffered injuries as a result of being attacked by two youths ...'. The physical findings should be detailed and quantified as far as possible. For example, say 'there was a 3×4 cm bruise on the lateral aspect of the left calf'. If possible, they should be illustrated with diagrams. All relevant physical findings should be stated, whether they are positive or negative. All physical findings which may indicate the degree of severity of the condition or the prognosis should be given. All relevant investigative results should be stated, whether they are positive or negative. The differential diagnoses at the time and the treatments given should be stated.

3 *Conclusions.*
An opinion of the condition of the patient should be given, and it should be clear why the conclusions were reached. State how far the physical and investigative findings support the history given by the patient. For example, you can say 'the injuries were compatible with those sustained by a sharp object such as a knife.' However, if you are unsure of the diagnosis, you must say so.

An indication of the likely prognosis could be given, if the doctor is confident enough to do so. However, the doctor should avoid making comments which could not be defended under cross-examination in court.

Report from an expert witness

An expert witness plays quite a different role to that of a professional witness. Expert witnesses are usually professionals who have special knowledge and experience in their field of expertise. In a personal injury case, the expert witness may be asked to examine a patient in order to give an opinion on the prognosis.

In medical negligence cases, the expert may be given documents and medical records relating to the treatment in question, and may be asked to give an opinion as to whether the treatment given was acceptable. The expert may or may not have seen the patient involved. Hence, whereas the professional witness offers mainly facts, the expert witness offers opinion.

Up to the present time, the lawyers representing each side of a dispute may ask the health professional for an expert witness report. The lawyers may decide to use the report or otherwise, and indeed to engage the same expert in future cases, depending on how favourable the report is to their client. As the expert witness fees are generally high, there have been incentives and pressure on expert witnesses to give as favourable an opinion as possible. Hence, there has been a general feeling that the expert witnesses have become 'hired guns'.

Lord Woolf's recent report highlighted the escalating costs of expert witnesses and the inordinate delays due to these problems, and proposed changes to the expert's role in future. The basic principle in Lord Woolf's report is that the expert's function is to help the court, not to advocate the case of the side by whom he or she is paid. In future, a court-appointed expert, or an expert agreed on by both sides, will be used more frequently. The content of the reports prepared for the courts will become more standardized. Whereas up to the present time, the expert is only expected to state his or her opinion, he or she will in future be expected to set out other relevant recognized body of opinion. The report itself must be internally consistent and logical. Further, it is likely that the court would be able to limit the expert witness's fees in proportion to the value of the claim in question.

An expert's report should include the following information.

1 *Introduction.*
(a) The expert's full name, qualifications and experience.
(b) A list of the documents which the expert has read in connection with the case.
(c) A summary of the facts and instructions given to the expert which are materially relevant to the conclusions reached in the report.
(d) A summary of the instructions given to the expert, and the purpose for which the report is written.
(e) Any literature or other material which the expert has relied on in making the report.

2 *Main body.*
A brief summary of the case, and the issues on which the expert has been asked to give opinion.

3 *Findings.*
The expert's main findings: this information may be gathered from the documents or the expert's own examination of the patient. If a test has been carried out by a person other than the expert, state who carried out the test or

experiment and whether it was carried out under the expert's supervision. Give the qualifications of the person who carried out any such test or experiment.

4 *Conclusions.*

(a) Give the opinion or conclusions on which the expert has been asked to comment. The conclusions should be logically deduced from the findings.

(b) Experts are often asked to give an estimate of the prognosis, often in numerical terms. The expert should strike a balance between being helpful to the court and providing a degree of accuracy which he or she is unable to justify. The expert should give an estimate only if he or she is prepared to defend it orally in court.

(c) If there is a range of opinion in the matters dealt with in the report, summarize the range of opinion and give reasons for the range of views represented.

(d) Give a summary of the conclusions reached.

5 *Ending.*

(a) State that the expert understands his or her duty to the court and has complied with that duty.

(b) The statement 'I believe that the facts I have stated in this report are true and that the opinions I have expressed are correct' should be included.

Appearing in court

Introduction

Most written reports by doctors and other professionals are accepted by the court as evidence and additional oral evidence is not required. This is especially true for relatively minor cases and if the report has been clearly and logically presented. Doctors and other health professionals are usually only asked to appear in court if there are disputes between the parties on facts or opinions contained in the report.

Doctors and other health professionals may be asked to give evidence in civil cases, in criminal cases or in the Coroner's Court. Small civil cases with claims of less than £50000 are usually heard in the County Court, whereas larger claims are heard in the High Court. Minor criminal cases are heard in the Magistrate's Court, whilst serious criminal cases are heard in the Crown Court. The type of court which a health professional will be asked to attend depends on the specialty in which he or she is engaged. For example, the junior doctor in the accident and emergency department will often be called to give evidence in minor criminal cases in the Magistrate's Court. Forensic psychiatrists are likely to be called to give evidence in serious criminal cases in the Crown Court. Forensic pathologists may be called to give evidence in the Coroner's Court and the Crown Court.

In civil cases, health professionals are usually asked to attend court by the lawyer who calls the health professional. In criminal cases, the doctor may be notified of the need to attend court by police officers. Alternatively, a formal witness summons may be sent to the health professional. The health professional may be called by the coroner to attend the Coroner's Court.

Again, it must be stressed that, if there is any hint of criticism of your own management of the patient, advice should be sought from the defence organizations or unions before appearing in court.

The prospect of being called to appear in court often proves to be both inconvenient and frightening for health professionals, and may lead to resentment at being called. One must remember two facts. Firstly, lawyers and the court are often very helpful to the co-operative doctor or other health professional, and are often prepared to do the best they can to minimize clashes with other professional commitments. Secondly, if you are unco-operative, you can be compelled to attend court by the issue of a subpoena. Hence, the best strategy is to be co-operative, and to let the court know of your commitments in advance.

Practical aspects of giving evidence

It will be helpful both to you and to the court if you understand the basic procedures of a civil or criminal trial and the formalities of giving evidence in court. Procedures differ slightly between civil and criminal courts.

Basic procedures of a civil trial

In a civil trial, the party pursuing a claim (e.g. the patient in a medical negligence claim) is the plaintiff. The party defending the claim (e.g. the NHS Trust in a medical negligence claim) is the defendant. Civil trials usually take place in the County Court (for cases involving sums less than £50 000) or the High Court.

The plaintiff's case
- The plaintiff's lawyer outlines the case in an opening speech.
- The plaintiff's lawyer calls witnesses of fact and expert witnesses. Each witness is examined by the plaintiff's lawyer, cross-examined by the defence and then re-examined by the plaintiff's lawyer (see below).
- The plaintiff's lawyer closes the plaintiff's case.

The defence case
- The defence lawyer outlines the defence in an opening speech—may be omitted.
- The defence lawyer calls witnesses of fact and expert witnesses. Each witness is examined by the defence, cross-examined by the plaintiff, and re-examined by the defence (see below).
- The defence lawyer closes the defence case.

There are then closing speeches by the plaintiff and defence lawyers and the delivery of the judgement.

Basic procedures of a criminal trial

In a criminal trial, the prosecution is represented by lawyers of the Crown Prosecution Service. The person being charged and tried is the defendant. Criminal cases are usually tried in the Magistrate's Court (for minor offences) or the Crown Court (for serious offences). Serious offences are tried with a jury consisting of 11 or 12 members of the public.

Charges are read out to the defendant and the defendant is asked to plead guilty or innocent. Members of the jury are then sworn in.

The prosecution case
• The prosecution lawyer outlines the case in an opening speech.
• The prosecution lawyer calls witnesses of fact and expert witnesses. Each witness is examined by the prosecution, cross-examined by the defence and re-examined by the prosecution (see below).
• The prosecution lawyer closes the prosecution case.

The defence case
• The defence lawyer calls witnesses of fact and expert witnesses. Each witness is examined by the defence, cross-examined by the prosecution and re-examined by the defence (see below).
• The defence lawyer closes the defence case.
There then follows:
• A closing speech by the prosecution.
• A closing speech by the defence.
• (The judge sums up and directs the jury).
• (The jury deliberates).
• (The jury delivers the verdict).
Items in parentheses are applicable only for serious offences tried in the Crown Court.

Basic formalities for health professionals giving evidence

• The witness is called to the witness stand.
• The witness takes the oath or affirms.
• The witness briefly states his or her relevant qualifications and experience.
• Examination-in-chief: the lawyer who calls the witness elicits the relevant facts or opinion from the witness. The written report is often used as the starting point.
• Cross-examination: the lawyer representing the other party challenges the witness's account or opinion given in examination.

- Re-examination: the lawyer who calls the witness clarifies issues raised in the cross-examination.
- (The judge may question the witness).

Practical points before giving evidence

- Ensure your clinical responsibilities are covered while you are in court.
- Know the case thoroughly by studying the relevant documents. Highlight essential points if necessary.
- Study your report to the court carefully.
- Rehearse giving an account of the facts of the case or the reasons for your opinion.
- Clarify queries with the lawyer who requires your attendance.
- Bring all relevant key documents to court. You may refer to them while giving evidence.
- Dress smartly and conservatively.
- Arrive at court on time.

Practical points while giving evidence

- Speak slowly and clearly.
- Look at the judge while you are speaking. Do not speak while the judge is still writing.
- Speak in plain language and avoid jargon.
- Do not transgress beyond your knowledge and expertise.
- Do not appear to be an advocate for one party. Your duty is to assist the court.
- Give an opinion only if you can support it with reasons.
- Do not contradict your written account without good reasons.
- Explain your opinion in examination-in-chief carefully and logically.
- In cross-examination, the lawyer representing the party will attempt to discredit you. Do not get angry, even if you feel provoked.

Reference

Access to justice: final report to the Lord Chancellor on the civil justice system in England and Wales (1996). London: HMSO, 137.

Index

Law for **Doctors**